Comprehensive Manuals in Radiology

Harold G. Jacobson, editor

Barry T. Katzen

Interventional Diagnostic and Therapeutic Procedures

With 114 Illustrations

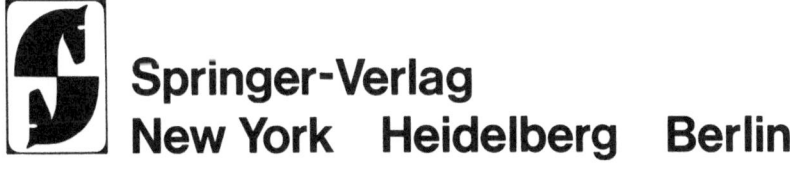
Springer-Verlag
New York   Heidelberg   Berlin

Series Editor

Harold G. Jacobson, M.D., Professor and Chairman, Department of Radiology, Albert Einstein College of Medicine (Montefiore Hospital and Medical Center), Bronx, New York

Author

Barry T. Katzen, M.D., Attending Radiologist, The Alexandria Hospital, Alexandria, Virginia; Consultant in Cardiovascular Radiology and Clinical Associate Professor of Radiology, George Washington University School of Medicine, Washington, D.C.

Library of Congress Cataloging in Publication Data
Katzen, Barry T
   Interventional diagnostic and therapeutic procedures.

   (Comprehensive manuals in radiology)
   Bibliography: p.
   Includes index.
   1. Radiography, Medical.   I. Title.   II. Series.
RC78.K3   616.07'572   79–28246
a

9 8 7 6 5 4 3 2 1

ISBN-13: 978-1-4612-6017-2   e-ISBN-13: 978-1-4612-6015-8
DOI: 10.1007/978-1-4612-6015-8

To Judi, Heather, and Lesley

Contents

7   Interventional Special Procedures   111

Appendix: Treatment of Reactions to Contrast Media   137

Bibliography   145

Index   153

Series Editor's Foreword

This monograph is most unusual. It deals in depth with the technical aspects of most special procedures used in diagnostic radiology, both interventional and non-interventional.

A large section is devoted to the various areas of angiography. As a preliminary, pre-angiographic orders, arrangements in the radiographic room, appropriate equipment, etc., are described, and similar information is detailed regarding the post-angiographic period. A discussion of the different types of catheters is most helpful. The various areas of angiography are described in depth. Every aspect of the technique is considered in detail. These include the type and amount of contrast medium to be used, the technical factors in the examination, indications, contraindications and possible complications. The subsections of angiography addressed include percutaneous axillary angiography, translumbar aortography, thoracic aortography, pelvic angiography, peripheral femoral arteriography and various types of visceral angiography with superselective techniques, e.g., left gastric artery, renal artery, coronary artery. Venography, including venacavography, adrenal venography and epidural venography, are well described. An appendix deals with the treatment of reactions to the contrast media.

An excellent section on angiography of upper gastrointestinal tract bleeding, detailing both diagnosis and treatment, is included, with consideration of the subject of embolization.

Angiography is only one of the major areas considered in this work. Other special procedure techniques are also meticulously described. These include arthrography in a number of anatomical areas, e.g., knee, ankle, hip. Other procedures considered are diskography, myelography, percutaneous transhepatic cholangiography, splenoportography, sialography, bronchography, hysterosalpingography, lymphangiography and methods of localization of mammographically demonstrated non-palpable breast lesions.

Direct interventional techniques are also discussed, including percutaneous lung biopsy, bone biopsy, non-operative extraction of retained biliary calculi and retrieval of intravascular foreign bodies. Transluminal angioplasty, using the Grüntzig technique (currently a popular subject), is also considered.

An excellent bibliography for each section discussed in the text is appended at the back of the book.

This unique monograph should be of significant value to a large number and variety of diagnostic radiologists. It is a particularly good "road map" and guide for all techniques, not only in angiography but in a host of other special procedures. As such, it serves as an important aid to the approach and diagnosis of many disorders, particularly vascular problems. It should be of great value to radiology residents and should be particularly helpful for those radiologists in smaller communities who do not have the opportunity to do a large number of many of the special studies discussed in the book. Thus, when confronted with the need to do such examinations, this monograph, which is well organized, lucid, complete and yet concise, should be virtually indispensable.

Although it is true that techniques in special procedures change quickly because of the rapid developments in diagnostic radiology, this treatise should remain important for a significant period of time.

Harold G. Jacobson
Bronx, New York

Foreword

It gives me great pleasure to be allowed to introduce this monograph. As the author states in his preface, it is a formal compendium of the various techniques required to perform many interventional radiologic procedures, those that are totally diagnostic and some that are therapeutic.

The increased involvement of radiologists in these procedures is evident to all. The astounding improvement in results over the last dozen or so years, largely due to such involvement, is also gratifying to one who has been involved in many of these procedures, especially as they apply to the field of neuroradiology.

As a teacher of radiology, however, it is quite difficult to easily and safely identify clear descriptions of the tried and true techniques that will allow a trainee, at whatever stage of his career, to begin to grasp it all, and to build a foundation for his further progress. These descriptions are scattered throughout the domestic and foreign literature of radiology, and such descriptions may have subtlely or overtly altered, possibly dangerously so, the original effective technique. This monograph should provide one-step easy access to the details of technique necessary for the performance of most procedures.

Obviously technique isn't everything, but it is an absolute prerequisite for success in both diagnostic and therapeutic procedures. The author personally has superbly amalgamated all the other ingredients that are necessary. He is bright, energetic to the point of tirelessness, conversant with the pertinent literature, amazingly informed in medicine and physiology, and in addition, highly skilled as a technician (and a superb teacher). All of these ingredients, and the fact that he intuitively possesses what I consider to be the two most important instincts of interventionalists, first, when to continue, and second, when to stop, make him an extremely valuable member of our radiologic community and our faculty. While functioning as a private radiologist, he continues to teach, write, lecture, and influence, and he has been quite instrumental in positively affecting the practice of radiology and medicine in his area.

I believe that this compendium will be a superb addition to the literature and congratulate all the contributors for their excellent work.

David O. Davis
Washington, D.C.

Preface

Recent growth in the role of the angiographer–diagnostic radiologist has paralleled refinements in image intensification and technical improvements in angiographic catheters, guide wires, and needles. The combination of percutaneous access, introduction of contrast, and high-quality imaging (including cross-sectional modalities) has allowed the radiologist to visualize virtually all internal structures.

Although noninvasive imaging is continually improving, numerous invasive imaging studies, including arthrography, myelography, venography, and arteriography, are routinely carried out in a busy diagnostic radiology department. In addition to diagnostic studies, the contemporary diagnostic radiologist may be involved in therapeutic procedures employing invasive techniques. This field, continually evolving and growing under the term *interventional radiology*, includes treatment of internal hemorrhage using angiographic techniques, biliary stone retrieval, percutaneous transluminal angioplasty, and percutaneous biopsy.

This manual describes the technique of various interventional procedures, both diagnostic and therapeutic, that are useful in an active radiology department. The text should be equally useful as a didactic source for initial instruction and as a handy reference for procedures less frequently performed. The "how to" approach is stressed, with little or no attention given to pathologic details except as they relate to technique. To guide the interested reader quickly to more comprehensive studies, references have been grouped by section at the end of the book.

There are probably as many variations of technique for a given procedure as there are individuals performing them. Improvements in technique are continually being made, and refinements may be made by the reader. Criteria for an effective technique include both safety and the success rate. Techniques included here have been found useful by the test of time, but are subject to further refinement. Many of these procedures will be replaced by less invasive methods of obtaining similar information. Even among individual contributors to this text, some variations exist, and these have been left, with justification for the differences stated. Where appropriate, significant alternatives are mentioned.

This work represents the time and effort of many contributors, since some sections required some subspecialty expertise. In particular, Robert Schneider, M.D., and Bernard Ghelman, M.D., contributed the section on musculoskeletal special procedures. Ray A. Brinker, M.D., and William V. Hindle, M.D., contributed to the section on special procedures of neuroradiology. Arthur R. Clemett, M.D., contributed to the section on cholangiography, Fernando Arevalo, M.D., the section on lymphangiography. Ira J. Green, M.D., contributed mammographic localization and hysterosalpingography. Michael H. Friedman, M.D., assisted with peripheral venography and with Marsha Racey, R.T., and Dara Basham, R.T., contributed the section on subtraction. Edward M. Druy, M.D., contributed to the section on interventional procedures of the genitourinary tract.

In addition to their significant contributions, Sacha Benjamin, M.D., and James Chang, M.D., deserve special thanks for their support of this endeavor. Hermina Benjamin, M.D., contributed medical illustration. In addition, Arthur R. Clemett, M.D., also a contributor, saw potential in a third-year resident and offered opportunity, for which I am grateful.

Although this text is a compendium of various technical details, certain aspects of special procedures are more difficult to teach. In particular, a certain "finesse" contributes to our individual success or failure rates, as well as safety. For me, this was a gift from Plinio Rossi, M.D., Rome, Italy, from whom most of my angiography training derives. This intangible factor, which I was fortunate enough to obtain in Rome, has served me well and I will be forever grateful. Finally, I apologize to my wife and children for the time that this project has taken from them.

Barry T. Katzen
Alexandria, Virginia

With Contributions by

Fernando Arevalo, M.D.
Attending Radiologist
South Hills Health System
Pittsburgh, Pennsylvania

Dara Basham, R.T.
Johns Hopkins University Hospital
Baltimore, Maryland

Sacha Benjamin, M.D.
Attending Radiologist
St. Vincent's Hospital and Medical Center of
    New York
New York, New York

Ray A. Brinker, M.D.
Director, Department of Radiology
Wayne County General Hospital
Eloise, Michigan

James Chang, M.D.
Chief, Cardiovascular Radiology
St. Vincent's Hospital and Medical Center of
    New York
New York, New York

Arthur R. Clemett, M.D.
Director, Department of Radiology
St. Vincent's Hospital and Medical Center of
    New York
Clinical Professor of Radiology
New York University School of Medicine
New York, New York

Edward M. Druy, M.D.
Chief of Computed Body Tomography and
    Special Procedures
George Washington University Medical Center
Washington, D.C.

Michael H. Friedman, M.D.
Attending Radiologist
The Alexandria Hospital
Clinical Assistant Professor of Radiology
Georgetown University School of Medicine
Washington, D.C.

Bernard Ghelman, M.D.
Assistant Professor of Radiology
Cornell University Medical College
Attending Radiologist
Hospital for Special Surgery
New York, New York

Ira J. Green, M.D.
Chief, Department of Radiology
The Alexandria Hospital
Alexandria, Virginia
Clinical Assistant Professor
Georgetown University Hospital School of
    Medicine
Washington, D.C.

William V. Hindle, M.D.
Attending Radiologist
The Alexandria Hospital
Alexandria, Virginia

Marsha Racey, R.T.
Special Procedures Technologist
The Alexandria Hospital
Alexandria, Virginia

Robert Schneider, M.D.
Attending Radiologist
Hospital for Special Surgery
Assistant Professor of Radiology
Cornell University Medical Center
New York, New York

1   General Considerations

Before the Angiographic Procedure

Patient Evaluation

This volume is based on the concept that a request for angiography (or other radiographic special procedures) is a request for consultation. Before seeing the patient in the afternoon or evening prior to any special procedure, the radiologist should first completely review the patient's history, laboratory data, and any x-ray examinations previously performed in order to determine what sort of examination should be done and to anticipate any examinations, i.e., venography or venous sampling, that might be necessary in addition to arteriography. Special attention must also be given to factors directly related to the examination, specifically previous allergy history and coagulation studies, including prothrombin time, activated partial thromboplastin time, blood urea nitrogen, and creatinine.

The patient is then interviewed, the examination(s) are described, the purpose of the examination is given, and the specifics of the examination and possible significant complications are explained. A pertinent physical examination should be performed and pulses checked at this time.

Informed consent should be obtained by the radiologist and witnessed. In addition, entry should be made in the progress notes stating that the radiologist has visited the patient, has explained the procedure and complications, and has indicated in general what examination is to be done. The puncture site of choice should be considered at this time.

Preangiographic Orders

Preangiography orders should be brief and simple. If appropriate clotting and renal function studies have not been performed, they should be ordered. An intravenous setup should be requested. The patient should be permitted nothing by mouth after midnight except water unless it is anticipated that the or afternoon, in which case a liquid breakfast may be given. For examination of the abdomen, and particularly if study of the inferior angiography will be done in the late morning mesenteric artery is anticipated, a laxative suppository in the morning, a cleansing enema, or both may be ordered.

Routine use of sedatives and analgesics "on call" is discouraged. Preferably each patient will be considered individually, and the degree of anxiety evaluated at the time of the initial interview. Usually diazepam (Valium) is administered intravenously in the special procedures suite because of its relative lack of side effects and because it can be "titrated" easily. Premedication with atropine may be considered for prevention of vasovagal reactions (0.5–0.8 mg intramuscularly). Premedication of pediatric patients is handled through the anesthesiology department.

Special Procedures Room

Prior to the patient's arrival in the angiography suite the radiologist should inform the staff of the specifics of the examination to be done in regard to film loading and any special drugs that may be required. When the patient arrives in the angiography suite, distal pulses should be marked on the skin: the dorsalis pedis and posterior tibial arteries for femoral artery punctures and radial and brachial pulses for the axillary artery. This will be a helpful reference during compression. An intravenous line should be present during angiography for elective administration of drugs and for treatment of any problems that may arise. Catheters and wires should be selected, and a water bath or steam should be available in case catheter shaping is necessary.

After the Angiographic Procedure

Compression

On completion of the procedure, after withdrawal of the catheter, the artery should be compressed for approximately 10 minutes unless significant hypertension is present; then compression for 15–20 minutes may be necessary. Extensive dressings and compression dressings are generally not used. Topical antibiotics may be considered. Generally a band-aid is sufficient for dressing. Distal pulses should be monitored continuously during compression.

Postangiographic Orders and Notes

After the procedure the radiologist should write a brief comment in the progress notes stating the vessels that were catheterized and the complications, if any, and give a preliminary report. Postangiographic orders may vary according to the puncture site, catheter changes, and complications. As an example, the vital signs may be checked every 15 minutes for the first hour, every hour for 4 hours, and then every 6 hours until the next morning. The puncture site and distal pulses should be observed each time the vital signs are checked.

Note: Before leaving the angiography suite the patient should be instructed how to administer first aid if the puncture site opens.

An order form stamp may expedite routine procedures.

Prevention of Thrombus Formation

Anticoagulation

Thrombus formation represents one of the most significant complications of arterial puncture and angiography, and numerous efforts have been made to prevent it, mainly low-dose systemic heparinization and irrigation, systemic heparinization, and coating of angiographic catheters and wires and other devices with benzalkonium chloride-heparin compounds. Considerable fundamental work has been done by electron microscopic and other methods that graphically demonstrates the results of prolonged catheter time within the arterial system. Complete discussion of this subject is beyond the scope of this manual, however.

Low-Dose Heparinization. Heparin 1000 units is diluted in 500 cc normal saline, which is subsequently used for intermittent or continuous irrigation of the catheter. This produces considerably less alteration in the clotting function than systemic heparinization.

Systemic Heparinization. In the method described by Wallace et al., 3000 units heparin is administered by direct intravenous injection, followed by irrigation of the catheter with 1000 units in 500 cc saline. None of the 525 patients who underwent arteriography manifested clinical signs or symptoms attributable to thrombotic arterial occlusion at the puncture site. Pullout angiograms of the puncture site suggested thrombus in 2.5% of 78 patients, as compared to an incidence of 50% previously reported. Primary disadvantages are that the method cannot be used in patients with bleeding problems and that the peak effect of heparin occurs at 30 minutes, which may be less than desirable in a short procedure.

Contrast Medium as an Antithrombogenic. Contrast material has been shown to be antithrombogenic, protecting the catheter from thrombus formation for significant periods. However, the total contrast medium required during a given procedure is increased, which may be a potential problem, although if the procedure is done properly, the total increase will be approximately 10–20 cc.

Outpatient Arteriography

In 1975 Giustra and Killoran reported considerable success in performing outpatient arteriography, in the standard manner, in a small community hospital over a 4-year period. After hemostasis the patient was observed in the radiology department for 2–4 hours, given instructions in administration of first aid and recognition of symptoms of arterial occlusion, and sent home to limited activity. Resumption of normal activity was permitted on the following day.

Of 100 patients examined, none was readmitted because of a delayed complication (i.e., after 4 hours). Two patients did develop significant complications, but these were noted within a short time after arteriography while the patients were still under the radiologist's supervision.

The authors describe the advantages of outpatient arteriography in a small rural community hospital; it may be of considerable value when hospital beds are limited and other social factors are taken into account, but there are significant disadvantages to its use in a large institution.

Photographic Subtraction

Subtraction is a photographic technique used to remove obscuring background detail and enhance contrast material on rapid serial angiographic films. This is accomplished by making a "mask" film from the first film in the series. The mask is an exact reversal of the film before arrival of contrast medium. When superimposed on a film with contrast material in the vessel from the same series, all background detail will be "neutralized." The contrast material then stands out sharply. Motion during the filming sequence is the major factor in failure of subtraction techniques. The detail on the mask must superimpose over the film with the contrast agent. Unless they match exactly, background neutralization is poor.

To produce a subtraction the angiographic series must be so timed that a film will be available without contrast material. This is usually accomplished by beginning the filming and and injection simultaneously or, alternatively, by programming a short injection delay. A subtraction mask is made by contact printing method, using the first film (without contrast agent) (Fig. 1a) and a subtraction film (Fig. 1b). Subtraction film is a special agent single-emulsion film developed for this technique. The use of regular x-ray film results in poor quality subtractions. A printing frame of contact printer is ideal for making subtractions. A mask must be made for each series for which subtractions are needed (Fig. 1c).

After the mask has been produced it is then superimposed over the desired film with contrast medium (Fig. 1d), and combination is taped securely together (Fig. 1e). Another subtraction film is then placed on top of these two films and exposed (Fig. 1f). In the resulting image the contrast material will be darker than any of the lighter obscured background. If desired, the contrast material can be made white as in angiography films by superimposing the unexposed subtraction film on the subtraction and making a print. This procedure is called first-order subtraction and is usually adequate to block out unwanted detail, although second- and third-order subtractions can be produced.

Rare is the angiographic series in which slight motion does not occur during the filming sequence; peristalsis and patient reactions to contrast material usually prevent production of a "perfect" subtraction. Often the whole film cannot be subtracted, but a selected area of interest can be superimposed successfully.

Epidural venograms, cerebral angiography, and aortic arch studies are enhanced when the subtraction technique is used to remove bony detail. Slight extravasation of the contrast agent in gastrointestinal bleeders can also be accentuated when subtractions are produced, as well as enhancement of tumor staining.

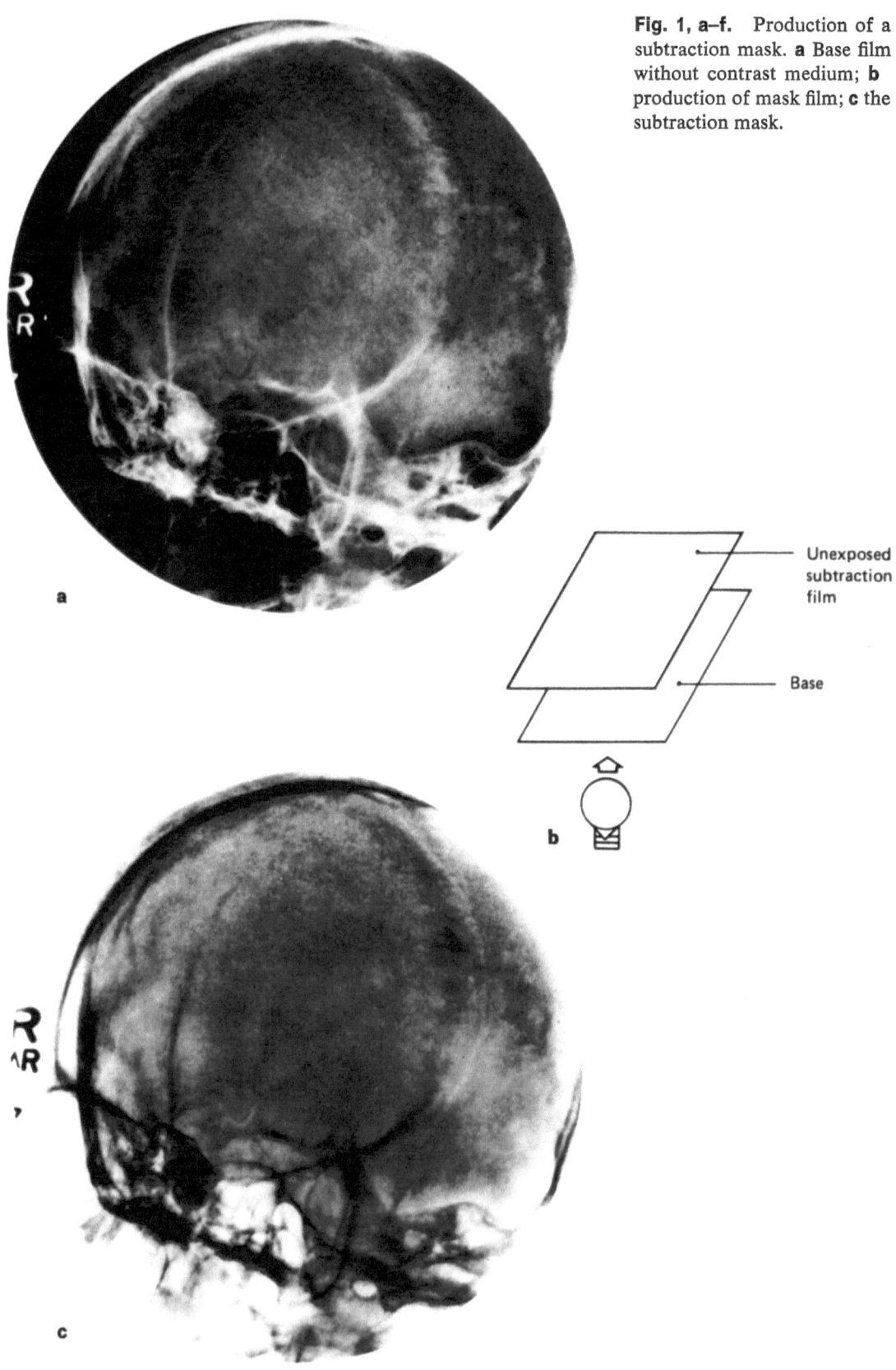

Fig. 1, a–f. Production of a subtraction mask. **a** Base film without contrast medium; **b** production of mask film; **c** the subtraction mask.

Fig. 1 (*continued*).   **d** Film with contrast medium but not subtracted; **e** production of first-order subtraction; **f** final subtraction product.

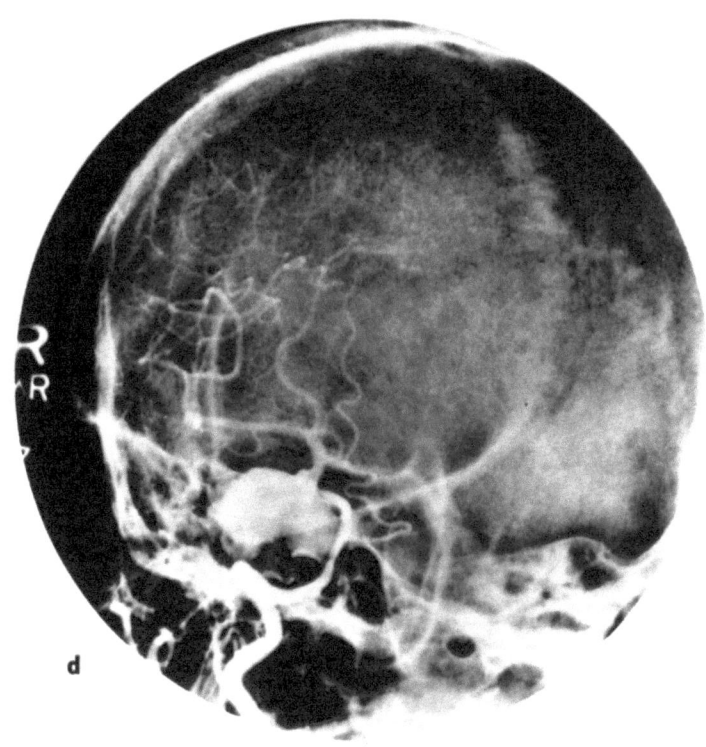

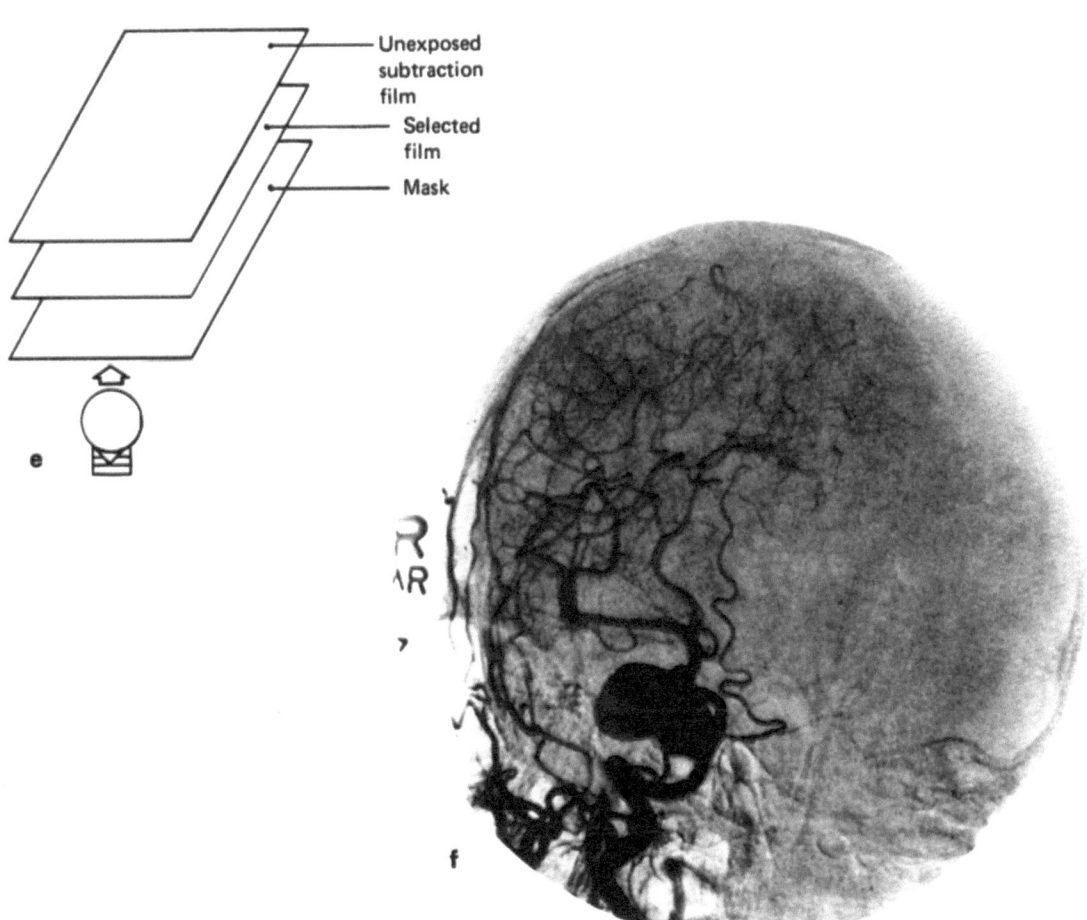

2 The Puncture

Check List for Starting the Procedure

1) Check fluoroscopy equipment
2) Start intravenous administration of diazepam (Valium) 2.5–10 mg as necessary. (An additional dose may be given prior to the first injection of contrast medium.)
3) Inspect tray
   a) Flush catheter
   b) Flush needle
   c) Double-check to see that the guide wire fits well in the needle and the catheter
   d) Ascertain that the tray contains appropriate contrast material and heparinized saline (1000 units/500 cc)

Local Anesthesia

Prior to preparation of the sterile field, both femoral pulses should be palpated. Both sides may be prepared with sterile antiseptic solution so that either may be used in case of difficulty in passing the catheter through one side or if a subsequent venous puncture is needed. After the antiseptic is applied the patient and operative field are appropriately draped.

The optimal point of arterial puncture is 3–4 finger breadths below the inguinal ligament in the common femoral artery. Once the point of maximum impulse (PMI) and anticipated puncture site are located, a small superficial wheal is made over the anticipated entry site of the needle. Approximately 1 cc of 1% lidocaine (Xylocaine) is applied over the PMI, and 3–4 cc is applied medially and deep and 3–4 cc laterally and deep. Aspiration should always be performed before injection of the local anesthetic. In addition, since the puncture will follow an oblique path from the skin entry site, administration of the anesthetic should follow a similar path. Excessive anesthesia over the PMI will make it more diffuse and the puncture more difficult. A small incision is made in the skin at the site of the original wheal to facilitate entry of the catheter.

The Arterial Puncture

Femoral Artery

Arterial puncture involves the same principles regardless of site. The technique described here applies specifically to the femoral artery.

The pulse is palpated in a straight line with the three center digits. With the fingertips in this position, not only is there palpation of the PMI, but there is two-point localization of the artery as well. While the pulse is gently palpated the needle is introduced at an angle of approximately 30°–45° to the estimated course of the femoral artery and *gradually* advanced toward the pulse until it reaches the periosteum, at which time the central stylet is gently withdrawn. The needle is then held with the fingertips of both hands and withdrawn very slowly. Adequate entry into the artery is indicated when there is pulsatile blood flow with good return coming from the needle.

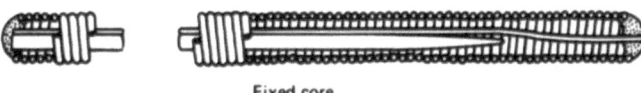

Fixed core

Fig. 2. Cross section demonstrating construction of standard guide wire. Courtesy of Cook Incorporated

The most common cause of unsuccessful puncture of the femoral artery in our experience is poor localization of the entry site. Most often it is placed too far below the inguinal ligament so that only branch vessels may be punctured. Generally 3–4 finger breadths below the inguinal ligament is adequate.

Disposable needles, which are extremely sharp, are available and allow increased sensation at the fingertips, providing easier passage through the arterial wall.

Guide Wires. Once adequate return flow is demonstrated (see previous section) the wire is introduced. The wire should always be advanced gently; it should never be advanced if resistance is noted. For general peripheral and visceral studies the wire should be advanced to the lower thoracic aorta. For simplicity, wires of similar lengths and diameters are suggested.

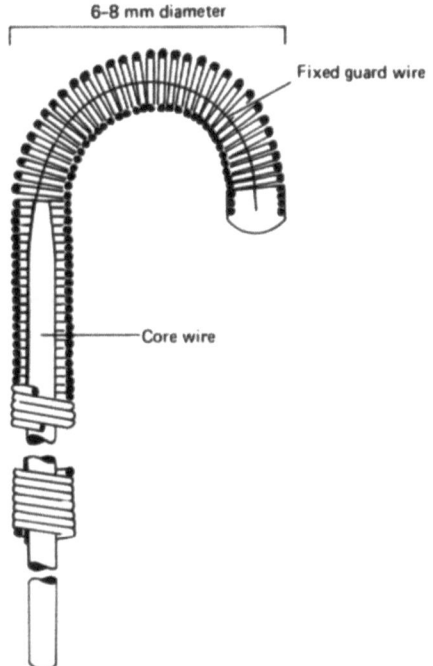

6–8 mm diameter

Fixed guard wire

Core wire

Fig. 3. Cross section of a movable-core ("floppy") J wire. The diameter of the J may be varied from 6 to 8 mm. Judkins MP, et al. (1967) Lumen-following safety J-guide. Radiology 88:1127

The guide wire represents the key to catheter angiography. It provides the means for catheter exchange and constant access to an artery, eliminating the need for arterial cutdown. In addition, the guide wire is used to provide support for the catheter while it is being passed into the arterial wall. Once access to the arterial system is obtained and the catheter is in place, the guide wire leads the way in tortuous vessels, after which the catheter may follow. It is of considerable value in superselective work; however, the guide wire is of greater thrombogenicity than most catheters and the amount of time the wire remains in the vessel should be kept to the minimum necessary. There are five types of guide wires:

1) Simple straight. This wire may be used in routine procedures in patients in whom tortuosity of vessels is not anticipated (Fig. 2).

2) J wire. This wire is extremely helpful in negotiating tortuous vessels; because of the curved leading edge it is much less traumatic than a straight wire (Fig. 3).

3) "Floppy" J wire. This wire has a movable core that allows the distal portion to become floppy and is useful in extremely tortuous vessels.

4) "Floppy" straight wire. This wire is particularly useful in venacavography and extremely valuable in superselective work. This will be explained in detail in the discussion of superselective catheterization. A floppy straight wire may provide the functions of all of the above (Fig. 4).

5) Recently, a variable stiffness guide wire has been developed which is "floppy," but can be stiffened by means of the handle used for the deflector wire (ref to deflector). We have found this to be quite helpful in doing superselective work as well as catheterizing tortuous vessels of the aortic arch.

Placing the Catheter. Once the wire is in the optimal position the operator applies mild compression superior to the puncture site with the left hand while holding the wire firmly

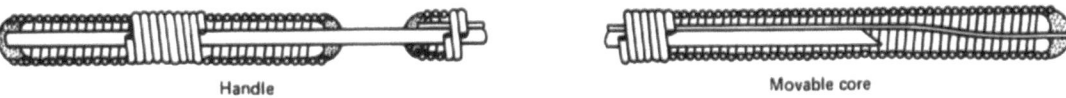

Handle   Movable core

Fig. 4. Cross section of a movable-core ("floppy") straight wire. Courtesy of Cook Incorporated

with the right hand. At this time the assistant removes the needle, wipes the guide wire with a saline sponge, and places the catheter over the guide wire and advances it to the entry site. Holding the catheter near the tip and simultaneously releasing the compression applied with the left hand, the operator advances and twists the catheter in the same maneuver, introducing it into the arterial lumen. (This is one of the critical points in the procedure: Incorrect introduction of the catheter may result in arterial trauma and continuous oozing around the catheter.) The operator gently advances the catheter farther while the assistant simultaneously holds and retracts the guide wire. When the catheter is in position in the upper abdominal aorta and the guide has been removed, the initial blood is aspirated and discarded. The catheter is immediately irrigated with heparinized saline. (Dilators or introducers may be used with catheters of ex-

tremely small caliber, curved catheters without tapered tips or mesh core, and at the discretion of the operator. In general, an introducer will not be required with a tapered-tip catheter.)

Catheter Irrigation. Irrigation of the catheter is extremely important in the prevention of clot formation. Two basic systems may be employed: continuous flushing (closed system), with or without pressure monitoring, and intermittent flushing (open system) (Fig. 5).

Continuous flushing is quite effective for end-hole catheters but less effective for multiple side-hole catheters (e.g., pigtail), since the bulk of the flow in the latter group of catheters will come from the proximal holes, leaving the distal portion more prone to clot (Fig. 6). The fact that it is a closed system implies that once the system is set up it is closed to external factors, particularly air. A variation of this may be used with a manifold

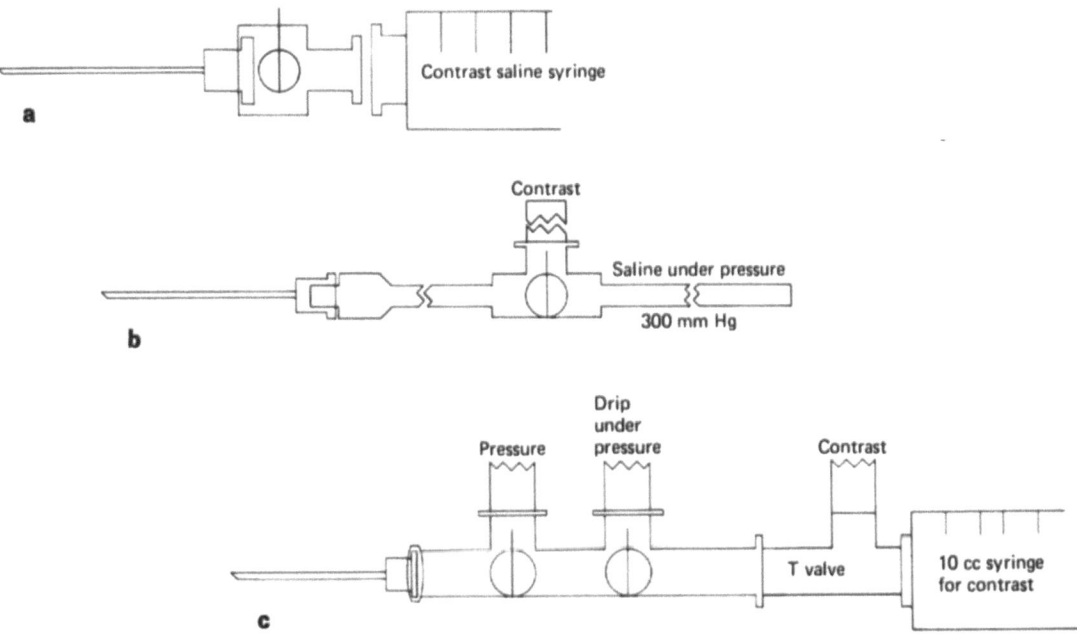

Fig. 5. Systems for catheter irrigation. **a** intermittent flush via syringe; **b** continuous drip, closed system; **c** continuous drip, closed system, with pressure monitoring.

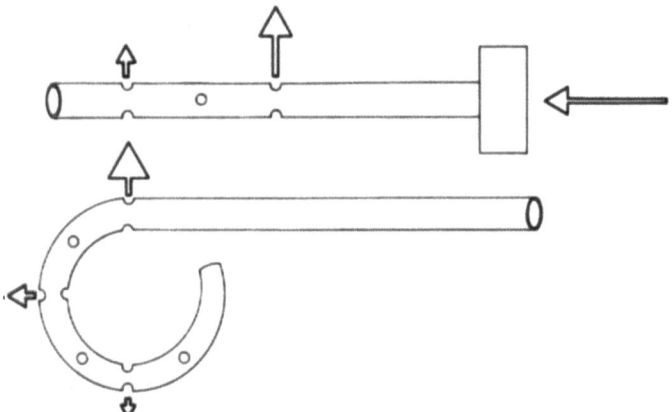

Fig. 6. Straight and pigtail catheters under continuous drip. Most irrigation fluid exits from the proximal holes with very little coming from the distal holes and none from the tip.

system of stopcocks, which will allow alternate pressure monitoring, continuous drip, and contrast.

Continuous flushing is of greatest importance in neuroangiography and coronary arteriography, in which small fibrin accumulations may have grave significance. We have found this system to be cumbersome for superselective work and prefer intermittent flushing in the abdomen.

Note: The more side-holes, the more readily thrombus develops.

Intermittent flushing is an open system in that the syringes containing contrast material and saline are continuously exchanged at the stopcock level, and the system is periodically open to the air and other factors. When this system is used, frequent aspiration (30–60 s), followed by flushing with fresh saline, is necessary; 3–5 ml heparinized saline is used. One should always be aware of the quantities of normal saline used, especially in patients with underlying cardiac disease.

Catheter Exchange. To exchange catheters the guide wire is advanced through the catheter to the lower thoracic aorta, and the catheter is then withdrawn slowly over the guide wire while the tip of the guide wire remains in the same position. This may be accomplished by simultaneous withdrawal of the catheter and advancement of the wire, or the wire may be advanced to the lower thoracic aorta and the position confirmed and maintained under fluo-

roscopic control while the catheter is removed. Once the catheter has been removed from the skin surface, gentle pressure is applied with one hand cephalad to the puncture site to reduce oozing and development of hematoma, while the other hand *secures* the wire. The assistant then, with wet gauze or nylon, wipes the catheter clean.

Next, the new catheter is threaded over the wire by the assistant. After the catheter has been advanced to the puncture site, the assistant holds the wire straight while the operator gently advances the catheter over the guide wire in a twisting motion, reentering the artery. If there is too much slack in the wire while the catheter is being placed in the artery, there is increased risk of kinking the wire and subsequently lacerating the arterial wall. After placement of the catheter the wire is removed; this is followed by immediate aspiration and irrigation.

Note: Multiple catheter changes may result in oozing of blood at the puncture site, in which case, introduction of a catheter one French size larger (e.g., a change from 6 F to 7 F) will generally stop the oozing.

Occlusion of Catheters. Occasionally, in spite of efforts for anticoagulation, catheters do occlude, sometimes immediately after insertion. For this reason, rapid aspiration of the catheter is suggested after the wire is removed. If blood is not returned from the catheter, the tip, which may be lying against the arterial wall, should first be located fluoroscopically. If it is an end-hole-only catheter, the tip should be repositioned in an arterial orifice and aspiration attempted again. While the angiographer is attempting this maneuver a high-pressure suction syringe is readied for use in case the maneuver fails.

If attempts at aspiration are unsuccessful the catheter is manipulated into a visceral vessel, preferably the celiac axis. A wire is then placed to evaluate the approximate length or site of occlusion. If it is relatively short, an attempt is made to pass a wire through the length of the obstruction. Other relatively "safe arteries" include the hypogastric arteries in the pelvis.

A second, safer, method is to exchange the catheter via a sheath. This is done by cutting the catheter through and through, placing a sheath over it, and introducing this into the artery. The catheter is then removed through the sheath and another catheter placed, leaving the sheath in place. This method is extremely helpful, allowing use of catheters of the same size even though the sheath has made a somewhat larger hole in the artery.

A third method is to use the catheter as a "guide" for piggyback passage of the wire into the arterial system, after which the catheter is removed. The new catheter placed over the guide wire should be one size larger to allow for the increased size of the hole in the artery made by the additional wire.

The Tortuous Iliac Artery. Not infrequently after successful arterial puncture the iliac vessels are found to be tortuous and to produce large curves in the catheter that affect the action of its tip, a situation that may present a considerable obstacle in superselective catheterization as well as in simple passage of the catheter to the abdominal aorta. Several methods are available to overcome this.

The floppy J wire is of considerable help in negotiating tortuous iliac vessels in which there may be numerous plaques. As opposed to straight wire, the tip of which may lodge in an atherosclerotic plaque, a J wire glances off these plaques and will advance more easily (Fig. 7).

A second aid is the floppy straight wire. When the tip of the wire becomes lodged on

a plaque or other site, increasing the floppy segment on the wire and continually advancing the wire gently create an effective J configuration inasmuch as the leading edge of the advancing segment is curved. Once this segment is passed into the abdominal aorta the catheter may be passed.

If these maneuvers fail and the wire will not advance beyond tortuous iliac vessels, a catheter may be passed after the tip of the wire is carefully fixed under fluoroscopy so that is not accidentally withdrawn from the artery. In this manner the catheter gains access to the arterial system, and the iliac artery may be "catheterized" by use of combined wire and catheter techniques. The iliac tortuosity almost always can be overcome with one of these three methods.

Percutaneous Axillary Angiography

The axillary artery has been widely used for access to the arterial system for selective catheterization. Reports of the morbidity of this procedure seem to vary; however, it is generally agreed that the transaxillary approach has a higher complication rate than the transfemoral approach. (Complications and prevention of potential complications are discussed at the end of this section.)

The right axillary artery generally provides easier access to the arch, while the left axillary artery provides easier access to the descending aorta for selective catheterization of the visceral arteries. Two ways to negotiate the arch anatomy are illustrated in Figs. 8 and 9.

Patient Positioning

Supine with arm extended and elbow flexed so head rests on palm

Technique

Careful palpatation will locate the artery in the axillary fossa *distal* to the humeral head. Local anesthesia is administered, as described previously, with 6–8 cc 1% lidocaine. After a small wheal is made, a 22-gauge needle is used to place anesthesia on both sides of the artery as well as a small amount over it. A

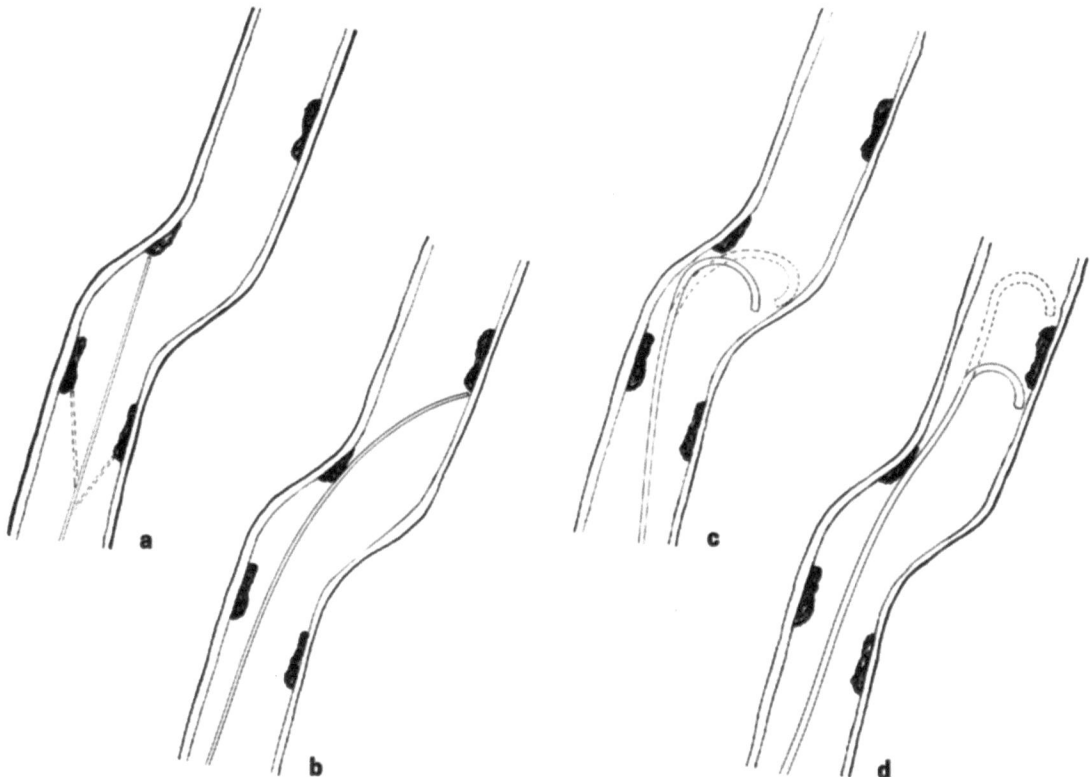

Fig. 7, a–d. Negotiating the tortuous iliac artery. **a, b** Conventional flexible tip guide may not pass through a tortuous iliac artery, depending on the number of angles and atherosclerotic plaques. There is some potential for dislodgment of these plaques and subintimal dissection. **c, d** The J wire more readily negotiates tortuous vessels, and with the additional use of a movable core, more tortuous vessels may be catheterized.

small skin incision is made, and an 18-gauge Seldinger type of needle is placed so that the puncture will be in the third portion of the axillary artery. (Disposable needles are much preferred to reusable ones because they are sharper.) Here the artery is more superficial than at either the proximal or distal course. The major advantages for puncturing at this site are: (1) The orifice of the anterior circumflex artery, a potential source of collateral flow, is proximal to the point of entry; (2) this portion of the axillary artery may be easily palpated and separated from the adjacent nerve fibers; and (3) there is adequate distance between the pectoralis major muscle and the puncture site to control bleeding.

After the needle is placed it is slowly withdrawn until pulsatile, free flow of blood is demonstrated. The needle is then brought close to the skin surface to accommodate the ana-

tomic course of the axillary artery. A J wire is then advanced approximately 5 in. *only* if the guide wire passes freely. The position is then checked under fluoroscopy since the wire may course easily into branches of the axillary or subclavian arteries. Molnar has pointed out that the vertebral artery can be avoided if the curved wire is passed into the innominate artery during a deep inspiratory effort.

In contradistinction to the transfemoral approach, in the transaxillary approach the catheter should be introduced only after the guide wire is successfully passed into the aorta. Attempts at catheter manipulation of a tortuous innominate artery may result in significant subintimal dissection and may have considerable import because of the close origin of the intracranial vessels.

After the catheter is successfully introduced, rapid aspiration and irrigation should be per-

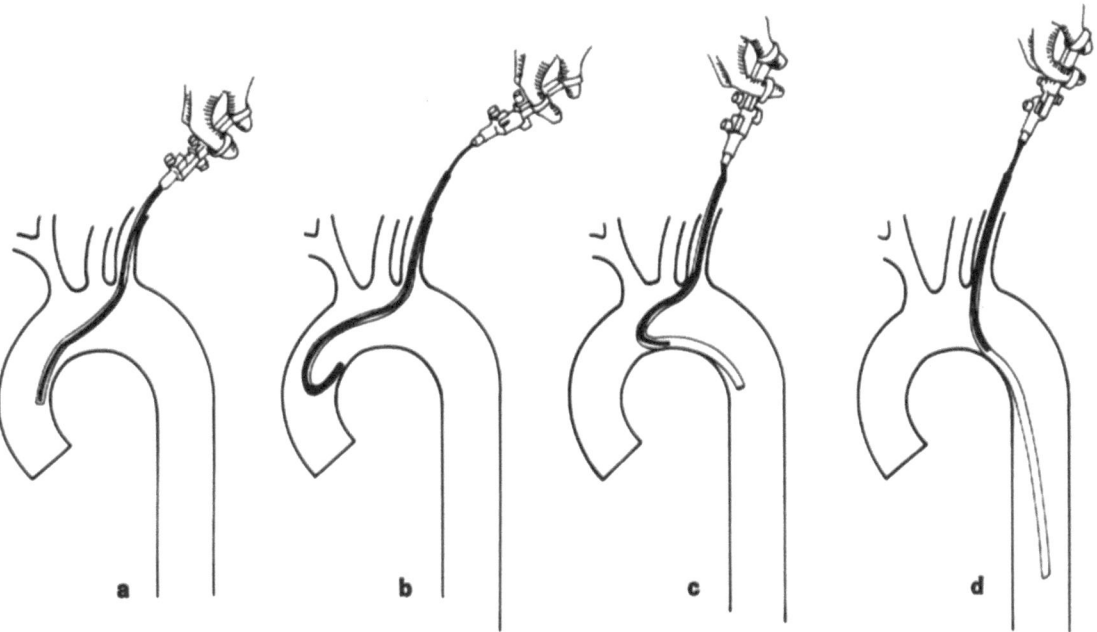

Fig. 8, a–d. Use of deflector system to place catheter in the abdominal aorta via the left axillary approach. **a** Deflector wire is passed to the tip of catheter in the ascending aorta. **b** Maximum deflection reverses direction of catheter tip. **c** The catheter-wire apparatus is withdrawn in the arch, and the catheter is advanced over the wire. **d** The deflector is released and the catheter further advanced.

formed. At this time, the radial pulse and the puncture site should be checked. It is also important that the catheter can move freely through the puncture site. Absence of the radial pulse, even when no signs of ischemia are present, should be an indication to expedite the procedure. Since complications appear to be somewhat related to the number of catheter changes, they should be avoided as much as possible during axillary arteriography.

Compression after Withdrawal of the Catheter

When the catheter is withdrawn a spurt of blood should be demonstrated through the arterial puncture site. The axillary artery is then compressed proximal to the arterial puncture site for 10–15 minutes, while the radial pulse is continuously monitored with the opposite hand. Constant monitoring of the color and temperature of the hand is helpful, and the axilla should be watched carefully for evidence of hematoma formation. As with other puncture methods, the patient should be in-

structed in administration of first aid and to notify the medical personnel immediately of any untoward events.

Complications (Fig. 10)

Thromboembolization
Hematoma
Brachial plexus (secondary to hematoma)
Pseudoaneurysm
Arterial dissection
Cerebral embolization

Preventive Tactics

High-risk patients should be avoided, especially those with
significant difference in blood pressure in the two arms, suggesting stenosis on the site of the lower pressure
severe systemic hypertension
severe obesity
extreme tortuousity of the right innominate and subclavian arteries (evaluated by preliminary chest film)

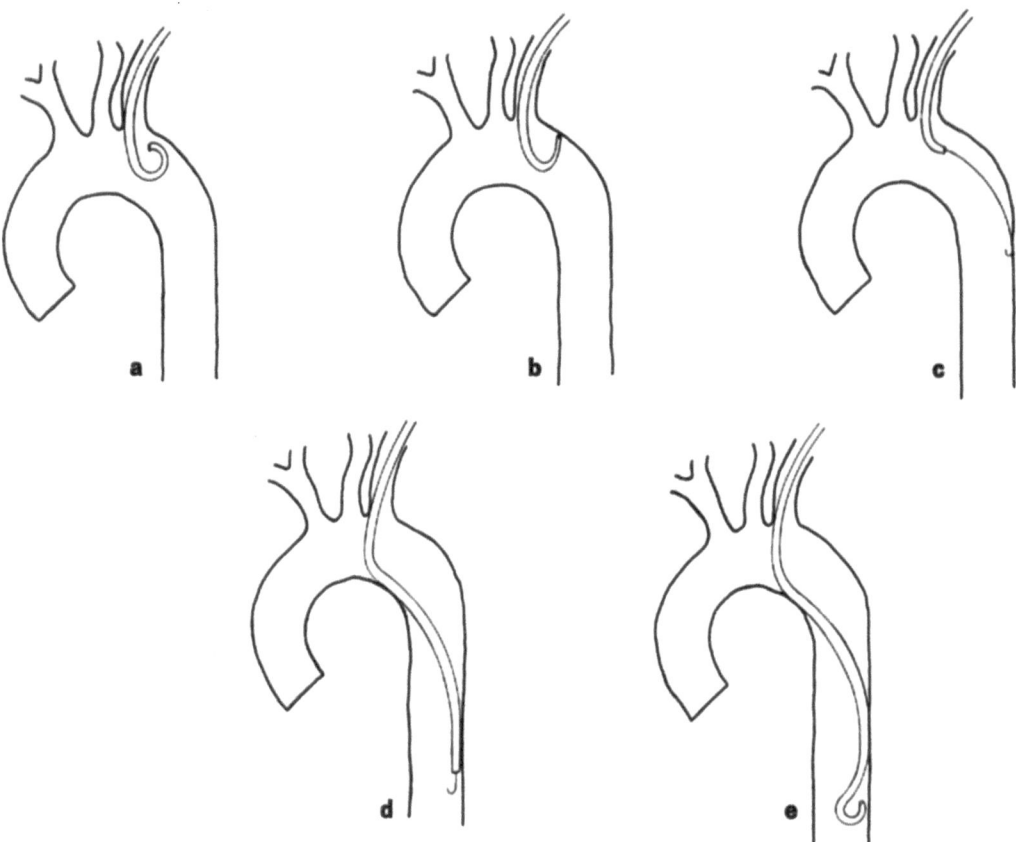

Fig. 9, a–e. Placement of pigtail catheter in the abdominal aorta via the left axillary approach. **a** Pigtail catheter is in place in the ascending aorta. **b** Slight withdrawal results in partial uncurling of the pigtail. **c** Guide wire is then placed into the abdominal aorta. **d** Catheter and wire are advanced. **e** Guide wire is removed with reconstitution of pigtail.

The Venous Puncture

In many respects, puncture of the femoral vein is technically more difficult than puncture of the femoral artery because it is a vessel of relatively low pressure that may occasionally lie posterior to the artery.

Induction of anesthesia is similar to that for arterial puncture; however, the lateral anesthesia is unnecessary. The key to successful femoral vein puncture is accurate localization of the arterial pulse under the digits as described in the technique for arterial puncture. If the operator always knows the position of the femoral artery, puncture of the vein is easier. In addition, with the femoral arterial pulse under the three digits, accidental puncture of the femoral artery should not occur.

The needle is advanced at a 30° angle to the approximate plane of the femoral vein until the peritoneum is reached. A 2.5–5 cc syringe is attached to the needle and the combination is slowly retracted, the syringe being gently compressed until blood is aspirated. During this step the patient may be asked to perform Valsalva's maneuver to further distend the femoral vein. The syringe is then removed, and the wire is placed into the femoral vein. Introduction of the wire and catheter is similar to that in arterial puncture. Fluoroscopy must always be performed during advancement of the wire, however, because of its frequent excursion into the ascending lumbar branches. In addition, more care must be paid to any resistance. Pain is abnormal during advancement of the wire, and if it occurs, advance-

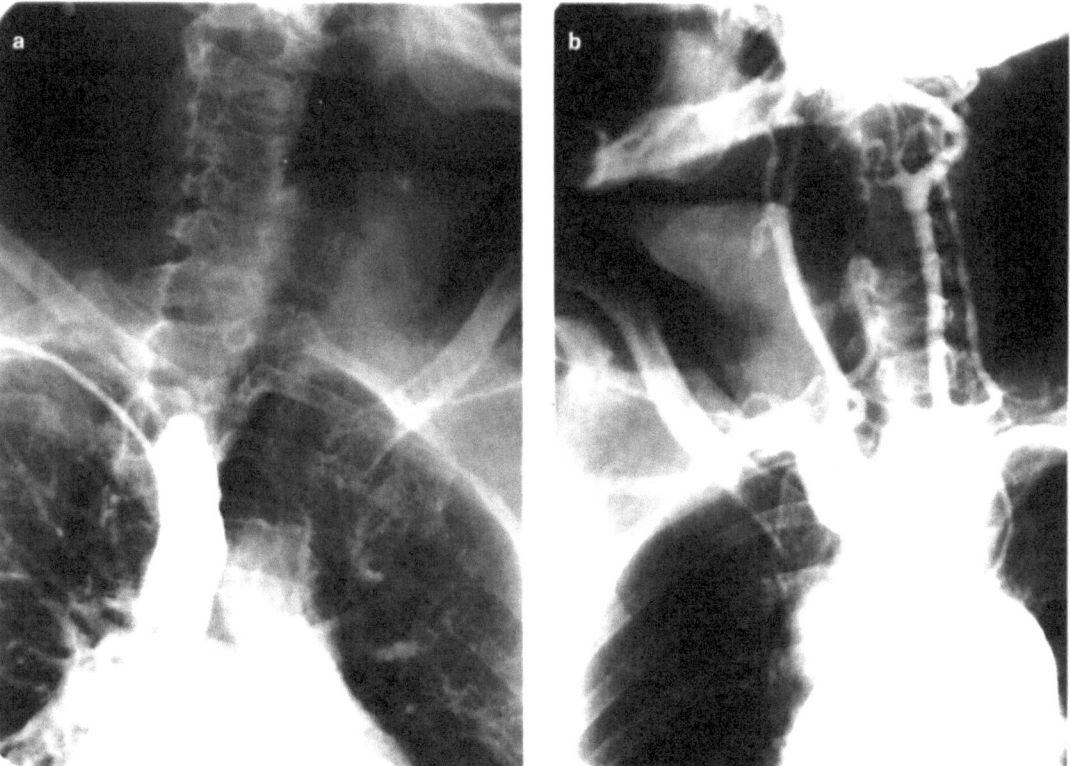

Fig. 10, a and **b.** Transaxillary arteriography. **a** After a difficult puncture there is subintimal dissection of the left subclavian artery. The appearance is one of obstruction. **b** Transfemoral arch aortogram shows relatively normal arch vessels, with some residual subintimal contrast medium.

ment should be investigated fluoroscopically. If difficulty is encountered after the wire has been advanced into the iliac veins, the needle may be advanced over the wire so that it is securely placed in the venous lumen during further manipulations. Use of dilators is recommended.

Introduction of a Sheath

In 1965 Desilets and Hoffman described a method of performing percutaneous catheterization using a sheath (Fig. 11) that would allow changing of catheters without a guide wire and, therefore, use of catheters with no end-hole. Since the original description this technique has been gradually modified (Fig. 12). It is used primarily in the venous system for introduction of Swan Ganz catheters; it is also used in pulmonary arteriography for introduction of side-hole-only (NIH) catheters.

In addition, the sheath may be an adjunct method of changing occluded catheters.

The prime disadvantage of this technique in the arterial system is that generally the sheath is one size larger than the catheter being used. For example, if a 7 F catheter system is used, an 8 F sheath will be required. Recently a thin-walled sheath system has been produced (Cordis Corporation) that allows free interchange of catheters of varying size through a sheath that may be irrigated.

Technique

Percutaneous puncture of the vessel is accomplished in the usual manner. A short wire is then placed (Fig. 12) and the needle removed, following which a short introducer is passed over the guide wire. A sheath is then passed over the combined apparatus and well into the vascular system. The introducer and wire are removed, and the catheter may then be introduced.

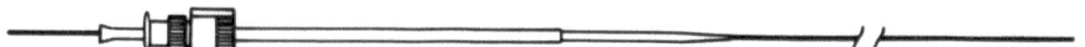

Fig. 11.   Desilets-Hoffman catheter exchange set. Courtesy of Cook Incorporated

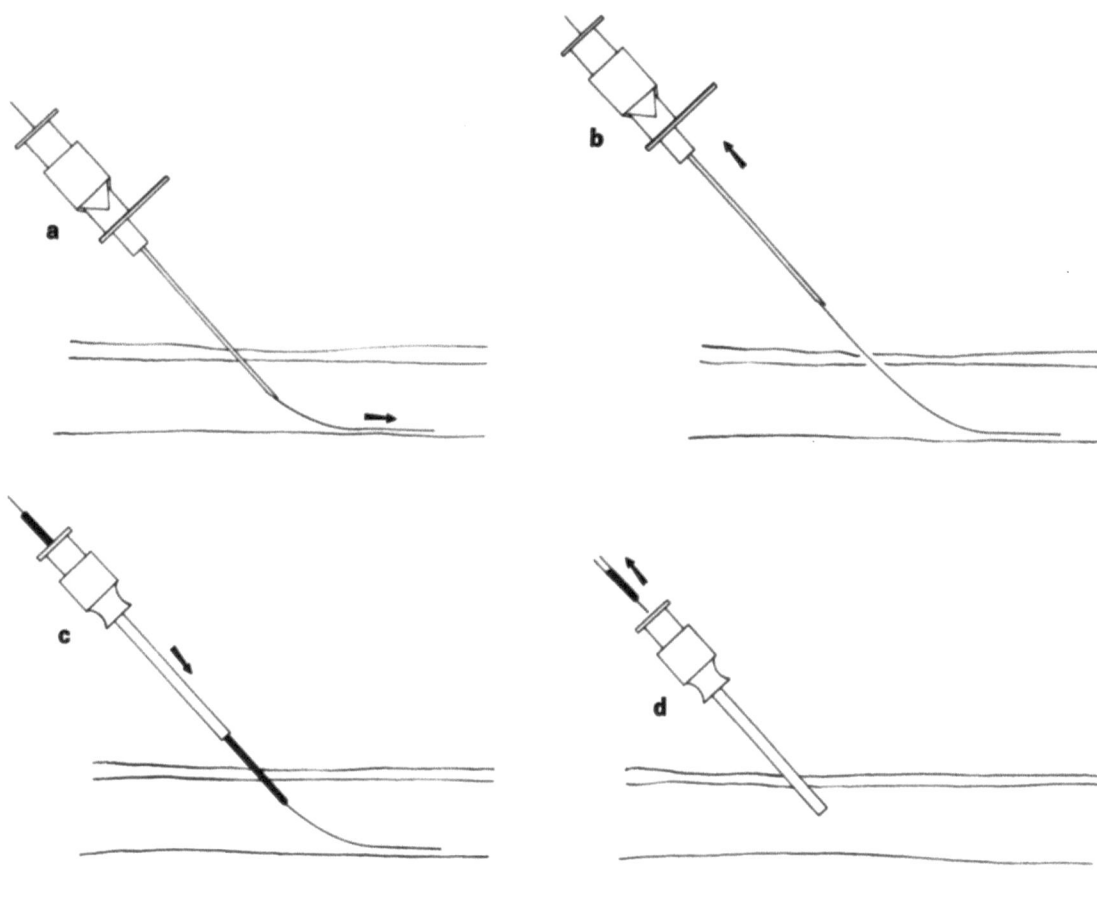

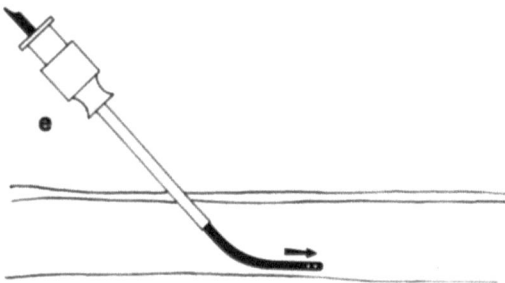

Fig. 12, a–e. Percutaneous introduction of a sheath. **a** A short guide wire is passed after percutaneous venous puncture by the Seldinger technique. **b** The needle is withdrawn, leaving the guide wire in place. **c** The introducer-sheath apparatus is passed over the guide wire. **d** The introducer and guide wire are removed, leaving the sheath in place. **e** The selected catheter is then passed through the sheath.

3 Arterial Examinations: Nonselective Studies

Translumbar Aortography

Translumbar aortography was first described by dosSantos, a Portugese surgeon, and associates, in 1929. This was the result of accidentally puncturing a human aorta on several occasions during lumbar ganglionic block and observing no complications. Subsequently the aorta was deliberately punctured, most likely so it could be used in parenteral drug therapy.

With establishment of a safe technique for access to the aorta, development of relatively safe contrast media, and subsequent development of vascular surgery, translumbar aortography became an accepted method of evaluating the aorta and the peripheral vessels of the lower extremities. This was the main form of arteriography prior to development of the Seldinger technique. As Rogoff and Lipchik have pointed out, although catheter angiography has largely replaced translumbar aortography, the angiographer should have this very valuable technique available because there are still definite indications for its use. In fact, translumbar aortography is again being advocated as the method of choice for evaluation of peripheral vascular disease.

The advantages of translumbar aortography lie in its relative speed and safety and its relative ease from a technical point of view. Disadvantages lie in the lack of selective and subselective capabilities and inability to place high flow rates through the sheath or rigid needle.

Purpose

To evaluate the abdominal aorta and peripheral vessels in patients with no palpable femoral pulses

Note: The transaxillary approach may be utilized in younger patients with peripheral vascular disease; however, in older patients, because of the high incidence of tortuous brachiocephalic vessels and the morbidity associated with the axillary approach, the translumbar approach is preferred.

Contraindications

Hemorrhagic diathesis
Increased prothrombin time (greater than 30% of normal)
Systemic hypertension with systolic pressure greater than 200 mm Hg

Equipment

18-Gauge polyethylene sheath with trocar
18-Gauge needle with Teflon sheath and central stylet (18 cm)
Venotube connector
Also available are polyethylene catheters that may have side-holes and are easier to reposition in the aorta.

Patient Positioning

Prone
Feet and lower legs rotated internally

17

Injection

15 cc/s for 3 s

It is our policy never to exceed this flow rate through the Teflon or small polyethylene sheath. Thus this is the usual sequence for aortography. It may be modified to reduce the flow rate for peripheral angiography, varying according to the type of equipment available for filming.

Technique

There are two types of translumbar approaches, the high and low. However, for complete abdominal aortography, the high translumbar is the one most often used (Fig. 13).

A distinct disadvantage of the *low translumbar approach* is that the site of entry is below the orifice of the renal and visceral arteries; the technique may be considerably more difficult in patients with atherosclerotic peripheral vascular disease because the anatomic location of this portion of the aorta is more variable than the upper lumbar aorta.

The skin entry site for the *high lumbar approach* is 2 cm below the inferior margin of the 12th rib and 8–10 cm to the left of the midline. After local anesthesia and a small skin incision to facilitate passage of the needle, the translumbar assembly is passed through the posterior musculature with a medial and cephalad course, being directed toward the centrum of the 12th thoracic vertebra superiorly. Once the needle tip has reached the centrum, it is slightly withdrawn and the direction of the needle is changed so that a more ventral course is obtained, glancing off the centrum (Fig. 14).

Note: Local anesthesia should be administered along the tract of the intended needle passage with a 2.5-in., 22-gauge needle. After this it is generally not necessary to repeatedly

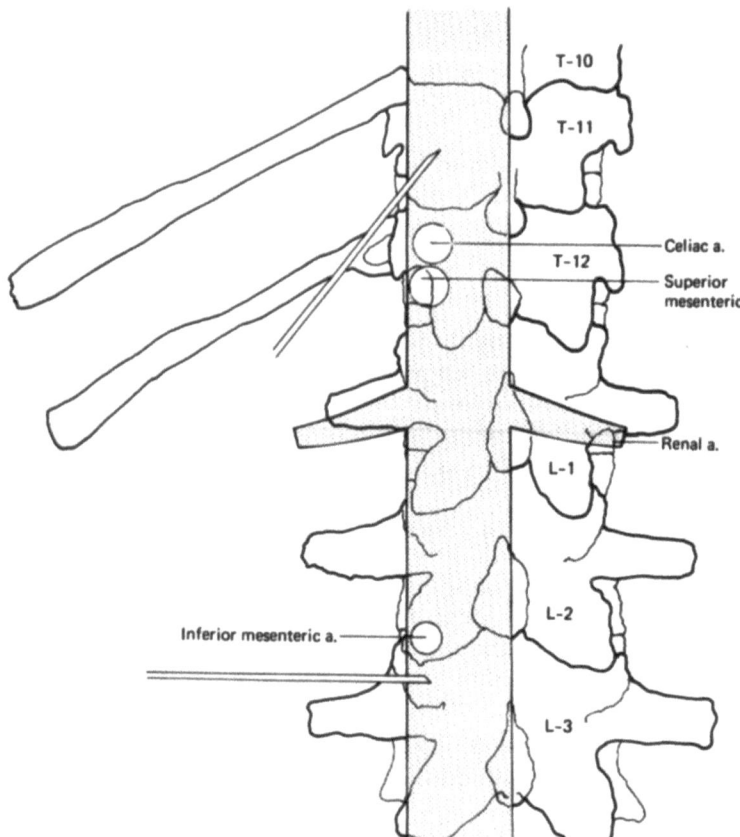

Fig. 13. Anatomic landmarks for translumbar aortography. *Upper needle* indicates the "high" translumbar approach, which is of benefit in providing complete evaluation of the abdominal aorta and study of the distal vessels. *Lower needle* demonstrates sites of "low" translumbar approach, which provides more limited information.

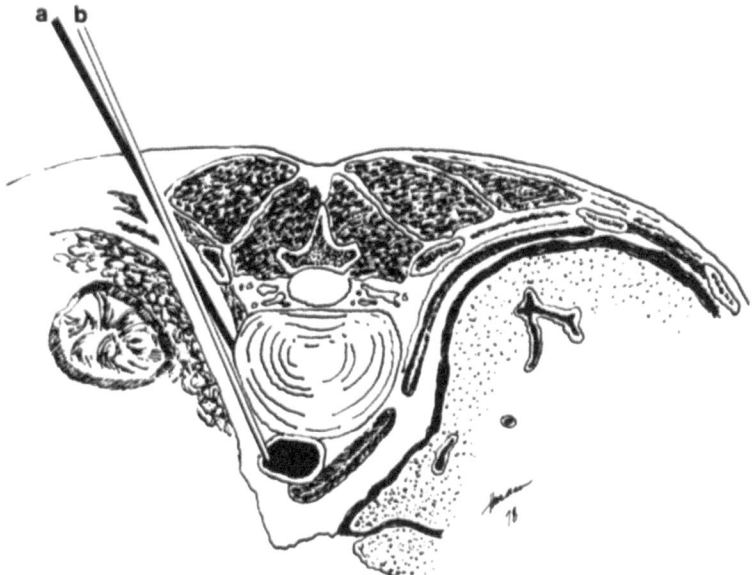

Fig. 14. Needle course in translumbar aortography. **a** Initial course of the needle until it reaches the lateral portion of the centrum is indicated. **b** Final course of the translumbar needle is seen after it has been directed toward the centrum of T-12.

place anesthesia along the needle path if a sure and steady hand is used in the needle passage.

The aorta is a thick muscular structure, and with careful attention, one can feel the aorta and the relief of tension as the needle passes into it. After penetration of the aortic wall, the apparatus is advanced slightly, i.e., 2–3 mm. The central stylet is then removed, only the sheath remaining.

When return of blood is demonstrated, the venotubing is connected and the sheath irrigated. When free flow of blood is noted, either of two courses may be followed: (1) A small test injection may be made to confirm the presence of the catheter in the abdominal aorta, followed by placement of a J wire with slight advancement of the sheath to insure its position well within the abdominal aorta. (2) A J wire may be passed immediately after demonstration of flow and the sheath then advanced. These latter maneuvers with the guide wire are extremely important to insure that the catheter remains in position during a power injection.

We have on occasion performed selective angiography by the translumbar approach, but this depends mainly on the closeness of the puncture to the celiac axis. In addition, for this purpose the high translumbar approach can be combined with use of a deflector apparatus.

Posttranslumbar Angiography

The patient is kept at bed rest until the next morning, preferably flat in bed for 4 hours.

The vital signs are as described previously, and as a routine precaution, hematocrit is determined 4 hours after the procedure.

Abdominal Aortography

Purpose

To demonstrate the central portion of the aorta and all branches by rapid injection of contrast material into the abdominal aorta

To evaluate parenchymal and venous phases on late films

Catheters

6 or 7 F straight with three to five side-holes, pigtail, or any other catheter that will accept 20–25 cc/s (Thin wall is preferred for high flow rates.)

4 or 5 F in children

Catheter position may vary, depending on specific interest. When interest is greater in the celiac axis, placement is made at T12–L1. For hypertension or peripheral arteriography the L1–2 interspace is preferred.

Approach

Predominantly femoral artery

Left axillary or translumbar approach considered if pulses in groins severely deminished or absent

Injection

20–25 cc/s for 2–2.5 s

The higher levels of flow rate should be used in patients with hypertension. A "low-dose" aortogram may be obtained with 20 cc contrast agent in association with high-grade Valsalva maneuver.

Film Sequence

10 films: generally 0.5–0.8 s delay

2 films/s for 2 s; 1/s for 3 s; 1 film every other second to run out (4 films)

General purpose of filming: rapid filming during arterial phase, slower filming for duration (10–14 s) to allow adequate visualization of later parenchymal and venous phases

Routine biplane aortography if equipment is available

Thoracic Aortography— Arch Aortography

A catheter is placed between the coronary ostia and the right brachiocephalic vessel with the pigtail positioned to open away from the outer wall. Generally interest is in only the early arterial phase and possible arterial collateralization beyond an obstructive lesion. In addition, the injection rate must be extremely fast because of flow and vessel caliber.

Catheter

8 (or 7) F pigtail or other 6–8 F thin-walled catheter

Injection

25–30 cc for 1.8–2.2 s

Film Sequence

0.2–0.6 s delay

3 films/s for 3 s and 1/s for 3 s

4 films/s for 3 s and 1/s for 3 s may also be used

Position

Visualization of the origins of great vessels and arch: Right posterior oblique projection optimal

In transient ischemia: Catheter proximal to origin of innominate artery; top of radiographic field at angle of the mandible; both oblique views

Thoracic aorta proper: Radiographic field lowered to include entire thoracic aorta

Dissecting aneurysms: Both oblique views; AP and lateral views if necessary

Pelvic Angiography

Catheters

For flush pelvic arteriography: Straight catheter with four or five side-holes; placed just above aortic bifurcation

For subselective catheterization of pelvis: Cobra catheter; used from ipsilateral or contralateral femoral artery. "Loop" technique may be helpful.

Injection

Above aortic bifurcation: 10–20 cc/s for 2–2.5 s

Selective hypogastric artery: 5–8 cc for 1.5–2 s, depending on size of vessel and position of catheter within origin of vessel

Film Sequence

10 films: 0.5–0.8 s delay

2 films/s for 3 s, 1/s to run out

Triple-Contrast Bladder Examination

Purpose

To evaluate the exact depth of penetration of bladder tumors (staging), bladder wall extension

Technique

Endovesical and perivesical air insufflation is followed immediately by pelvic arteriography. Pelvic arteriography is preferred to unilateral selective hypogastric arteriography because it allows comparison between both sides. Bilateral simultaneous selective hypogastric arteriography will give better detail, but sometimes it might require too much time, and part of the insufflated perivesical air could therefore be lost.

1) Perivesical gas insufflation. An indwelling Foley catheter is inserted and the bladder emptied. The patient is placed in the Trendelenburg position if possible, with the table tilted about 15°. The suprapubic area is prepared. Anesthesia of the suprapubic area is obtained by injecting lidocaine 1% at a point 3 cm on either side of the midline. Puncture is made with a 19-gauge 4-in. spinal needle directed posteromedially beneath the superior pubic ramus on either side (under fluoroscopy). A total of 250–300 cc air or oxygen is injected under fluoroscopy into the perivesical space. The needles are removed. The patient is rotated slowly through 360° in order to distribute the air evenly about the bladder; usually this rotation requires 5 min. The patient is returned to the horizontal position, 100–200 cc air is instilled into the bladder, and the indwelling Foley catheter is clamped.

2) Perineal approach to perivesical insufflation. With the patient supine, air is introduced into the bladder until there is an urge to void (200–300 cc). The Foley catheter is clamped. The patient flexes the knees and legs, which are spread apart. The operator introduces a finger into the rectum, and with a 19-gauge 4-in. spinal needle places a puncture in the middle of the perineum. Guided by the finger in the rectum the needle is directed to the right, lateral to the prostate in males, just distal to the bladder neck, and 200 cc gas is injected. The same procedure is repeated on the left side. Five minutes is allowed for the gas to diffuse.

Arteriography. This procedure must be done quickly because of resorption of air. The Seldinger technique is used to introduce a no. 6 or 7 straight catheter with multiple sideholes. The catheter is placed above the aortic bifurcation. One film is exposed for subtraction, and 40 ml of 76% contrast is injected over 2–3 s. An AP view is filmed with the tub vertical or 15° caudad and the patient supine. Film up to 14 s. An oblique view is seldom necessary. Selective hypogastric artery injections are helpful.

Note: In our experience this technique has been highly accurate in detecting extravesical extension of tumor, which may have significance in planning of therapy.

Peripheral (Femoral) Arteriography

In routine peripheral arteriography the abdominal aorta and all levels peripherally should be studied. This may be done with a single injection or two separate injections, depending on the size of the patient and the equipment available. If separate aortography is necessary the technique may be done as described in the preceding section.

On occasion only the femoral artery may be injected, a needle or sheath being used; however, simultaneous bilateral studies are preferred, generally by injection of contrast medium at the aortic bifurcation.

The study should not be considered complete until there is adequate demonstration of all vessels, and in cases of obstruction, adequate demonstration of collateralization. The trifurcation of the popliteal arteries and runoff vessels to the ankles and feet should be demonstrated.

Intraarterial Use of Lidocaine in Peripheral Angiography

Reports of double-blind studies involving intraarterial use of lidocaine for analgesia in peripheral arteriography seem to document its effectiveness in relief of pain. (One criticism of this study may be the use of significant amounts of meperidine [Demerol] and pento-barbital [Nembutal] for premedication.)

Two techniques have been advocated, one utilizing injection of lidocaine prior to injection of contrast material and the second utilizing lidocaine mixed with the contrast agent in the injector. No clear difference in results has been demonstrated.

1) Lidocaine 2%, 4 cc/50 cc contrast medium, given prior to injection
2) Lidocaine 2% mixed with contrast material in a ratio of 1:10 by volume

Although some controversy still exists, we have utilized the second method and believe it to be beneficial in relief of pain.

Catheter

Simple straight 5–7 F catheter with side-holes

Injection

Above the bifurcation, 8–12 cc for 7–8 s, a good starting point

Injection rates and film sequence will vary according to flow, and imaging equipment. A long injection (over 7–8 s) gives additional latitude in setting up film sequence, and reduces the margin of error.

Film Sequence

(for moving Spectrum table with four sequential positions)

Usually 16 films loaded consecutively, with brief interval (1–1.5 s) to move table
Generally 2 films/s for 2 s or 1/s for 3 s in pelvis with 1-s delay
1/s filming for remainder of films

The time between each position may be varied at the control panel. In addition, the number of films of each position may be varied. Preliminary timing of the flow of contrast medium to the knee may be made under fluoroscopic control. If a significant flow difference is demonstrated in each extremity a selective common iliac injection may be utilized.

Film sequence may be computed after timing the flow of contrast agent from the bifurcation to the knee. Specifics of timing will vary according to what equipment is available—moving table, long-length changer, etc. Our routine is to perform biplane aortography followed by peripheral arteriography, starting with top of the field at the iliac crest.

Note: The entire procedure described above may be performed by manual movement of the table and loading the film changer with empty slots during the period of movement.

4 Arterial Examinations: Selective Studies

Visceral Angiography

Prior to attempting any form of angiography, one must know the specific vascular anatomy and variations. Complete discussion is beyond the scope of this text; however, when appropriate, it will be demonstrated.

Catheter

Preshaped cobra 6.3 F (braided or nonbraided, with or without torque control) (Figs. 15 and 16)
C catheter

The first is the most widely applicable catheter for both selective and superselective work. In addition, a size-compatible group of preshaped subselective catheters is available (see Fig. 19). Occasionally the second may be useful; however, this shape is poorly suited for subselective work, and a deflector can transform a cobra into a C shape for entry into the celiac and superior mesenteric arteries. A single side-hole is helpful in preventing catheter "whip" during injection. Catheters without side-holes are needed for superselective work to avoid undesired reflux.

Injection

Celiac trunk: 50 cc, 8–12 cc/s
Superior mesenteric artery: 50 cc, 8–12 cc/s
Inferior mesenteric artery: 12–20 cc, 3–5 cc/s
Splenic artery: up to 25 cc, 6–8 cc/s
Common hepatic artery: 30–40 cc, 6–8 cc/s

Left gastric artery: 12–20 cc, 2–5 cc/s
Gastroduodenal artery: 12–20 cc, 3–5 cc/s

In suspected portal hypertension total vol-

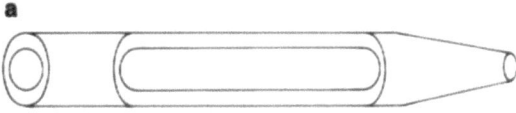
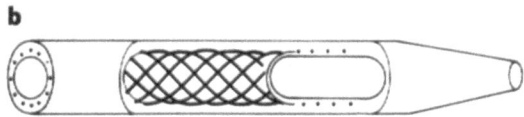

Fig. 15, a and **b.** Catheter construction. **a** Standard nonbraided catheter is shown. **b** Stainless steel braid provides torque control, avoiding catheter whip. Courtesy of Cook Incorporated

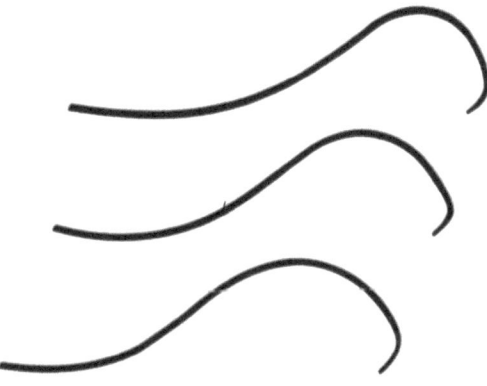

Fig. 16. Standard cobra preshaped visceral catheters. The secondary curve varies to accommodate aortas of differing size. Courtesy of Cook Incorporated

ume should be increased in the superior mesenteric and splenic arteries to 60–80 cc.

Note: These flow rates and times represent only a rough guideline and have to be evaluated individually in regard to vessel size and pathologic changes and in conjunction with the use of pharmacoangiography.

Film Sequence

15 films: 0.5–0.8 s delay

2 films/s for 3 s, 1/s for 3 s; and 1 film every other second or every third second to run out

Filming to 18–24 s routinely

In suspected portal hypertension, filming extended to 25–30 or longer as necessary

Determining Position of the Catheter Tip

After placing the catheter in the abdominal aorta, one places the T12–L1 interspace in the radiographic field, counting up from the lum-

bosacral junction. Once the desired field is attained, moving the patient (table) should be avoided, in order to keep landmarks in the fluoroscopic field constant.

To determine whether the tip is directed anteriorly or posteriorly the catheter is rotated clockwise at the groin and its tip observed (Fig. 17). If the catheter tip moves in the same direction, it is anterior; if it moves in the opposite direction, it is posterior.

Visual and tactile senses must be developed so that the catheter tip can be seen and felt as it reaches an aortic branch. When this movement of the tip in an orifice is sensed a small test injection is made for identification.

Catheterization of the Celiac Axis

The celiac artery most commonly originates from the aorta at the T12–L1 interspace, very often over the left pedicle of T-12. Therefore, when the orifice is being sought, movement of the catheter tip should be limited to this area. A common error of the novice in angiography is to "seek" over too large an area. Any identified vessels (e.g., or superior mesen-

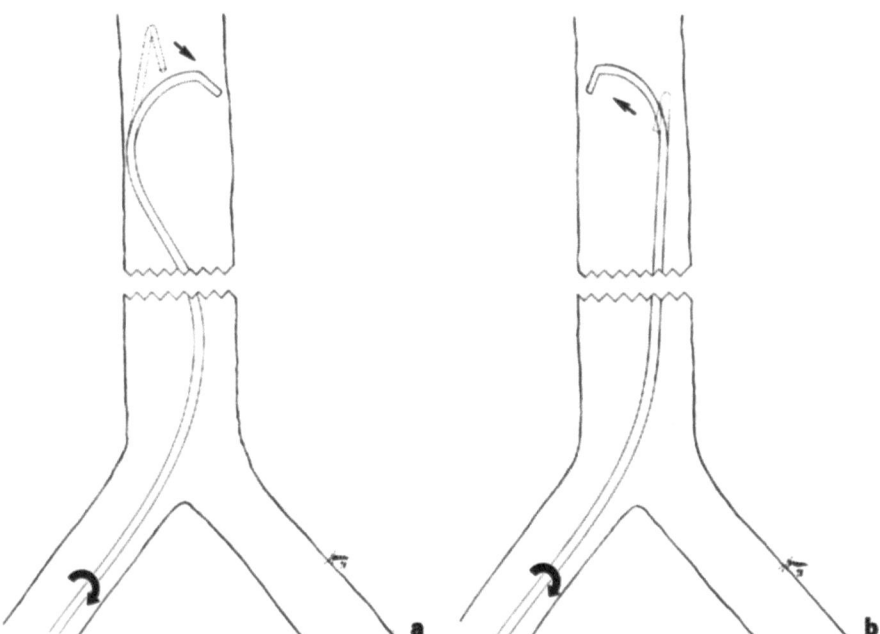

Fig. 17, a and **b.**   Determining position of the catheter tip. **a** If the tip is *anterior*, rotation of the catheter clockwise at the groin will move the tip toward the patient's left. **b** If the tip is *posterior*, rotation of the catheter clockwise at the groin will move the tip toward the patient's right.

teric artery should be used to aid in localization of landmarks.

Once the catheter is at the orifice of the celiac artery it is simply advanced. The catheter tip should be 1.5–2.0 cm within the celiac artery to avoid reflux into the aorta. A test injection, under fluoroscopy, may be made to insure adequate placement and to avoid the necessity for repeated attempts at placement.

If the catheter will not advance into the celiac artery from its origin, the artery may be stenosed, although the most likely reason is that the celiac artery is directed downward at too great an angle to accommodate the secondary curve of the cobra catheter. A floppy J or floppy straight wire may be passed through the catheter further into the celiac artery, over which the catheter may be advanced. A variable stiffness wire may also be used, as well as a deflector apparatus if other maneuvers do not work.

This problem may also be resolved with catheter changes, specifically to a C catheter. However, this shape has the decided disadvantage of restricting superselective work.

The Loop Technique in Visceral Angiography

Since the original descriptions of the formation of loop-shaped secondary curves of catheters for left gastric artery catheterization (using predominately polyurethane catheters) by Waltman, we have adapted the concept to polyethylene catheters and have eliminated the need for preliminary shaping, taking advantage of the patient's arterial or venous anatomy. The important concept of the loop technique is that the direction of the tip of the catheter is reversed by 180°. This fundamental concept may be applied in virtually any situation in which the desired catheter direction is 180° from the existing catheter position. Advantages over previous techniques are: (1) Preshaping is not necessary, (2) deflectors are not necessary, and (3) catheter changes are avoided. This technique has been successfully applied to both the arterial and venous system.

The catheter used is a preshaped polyethylene cobra (6.3 F Cook) catheter. The catheter is advanced into a large vessel, pref-

erably the main trunk of the vessel to be catheterized, and further advanced distal to the branch to be selectively catheterized. Continuous advancement of the catheter at the puncture site after the tip will not move any further results in formation of a loop in the aorta. With formation of the loop, simultaneous 180° reversal of the direction of the tip occurs, at which time all motions are reversed; advancing the catheter in the groin will result in retraction of the catheter tip and vice versa. This technique was originally described with coaxial systems and with catheters preshaped with heat. However, preshaping is no longer necessary, the looping being done entirely within the abdominal aorta once the standard cobra catheter is in place.

Although this technique was originally described in the arterial tree, we have also used it in the venous system, specifically for catheterization of the left adrenal vein (Fig. 18), in which we have used it successfully and without difficulty in over 50 consecutive cases. Since the basic catheter used for the right adrenal vein is the same cobra catheter (without the loop), this has reduced catheter time, eliminating the need for catheter change.

This technique has been successfully employed in catheterization of the (1) left gastric artery, (2) right hepatic originating from the superior mesenteric artery, (3) inferior pancreaticoduodenal artery, (4) cephalad-directed common hepatic or splenic artery, (5) ipsilateral hypogastric artery, and (6) left adrenal vein. In addition, when occasionally the catheter tip will not advance beyond the bifurcation of the celiac axis, employment of the loop technique will permit selective catheterization of either the common hepatic or the splenic artery.

The loop technique is easily taught to residents and fellows and represents a rapid method of subselective catheterization that avoids multiple guide wires and catheter changes.

Superselective Angiography

Superselective catheterization has come to have both diagnostic and therapeutic significance. Superselective catheterization of the ves-

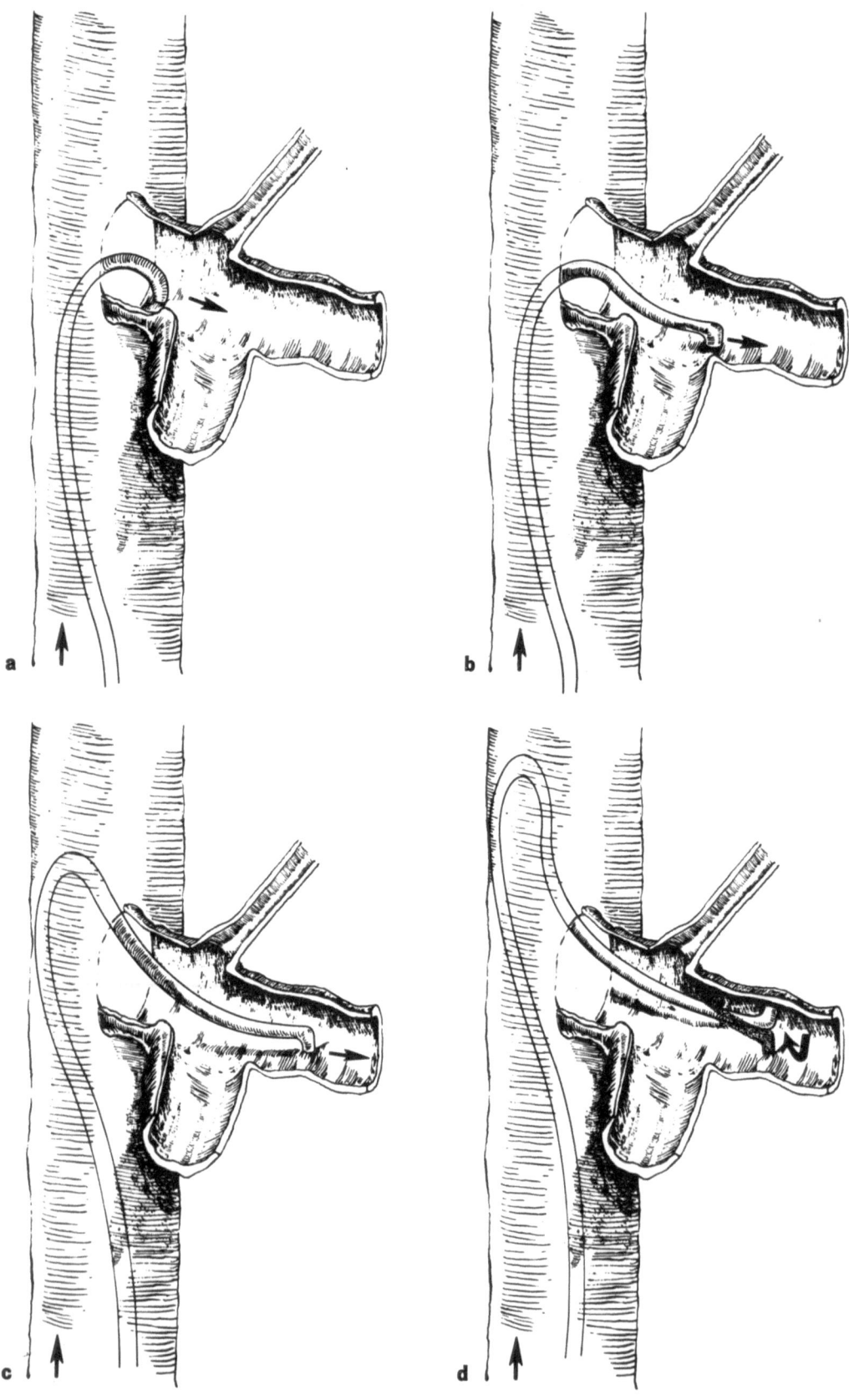

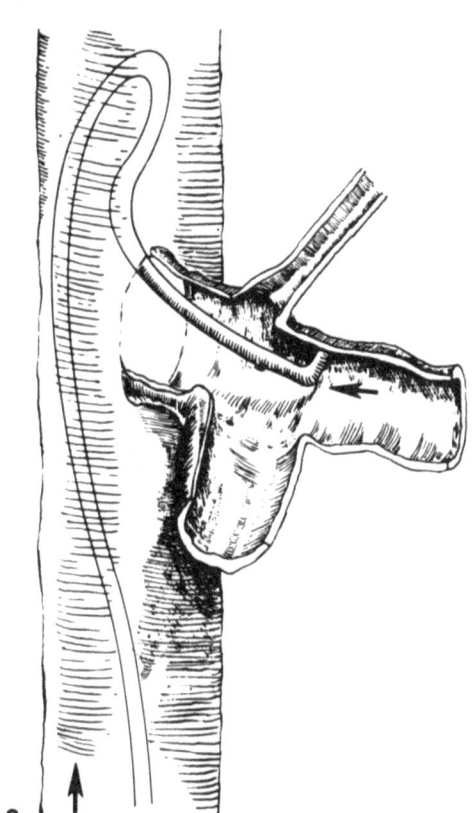

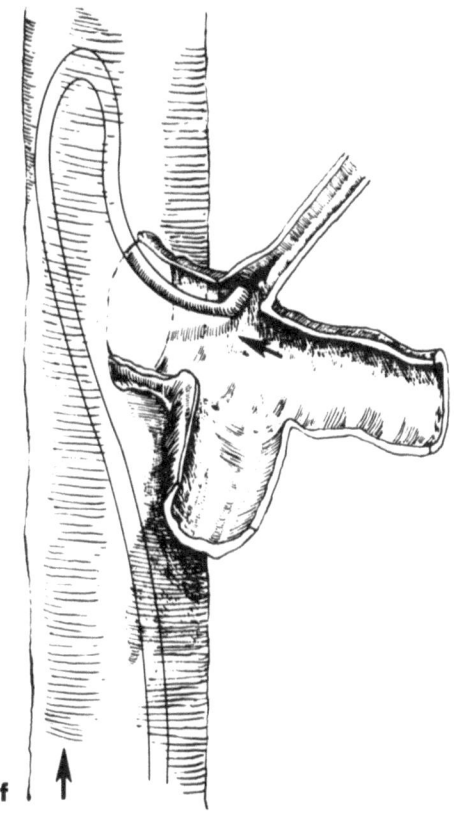

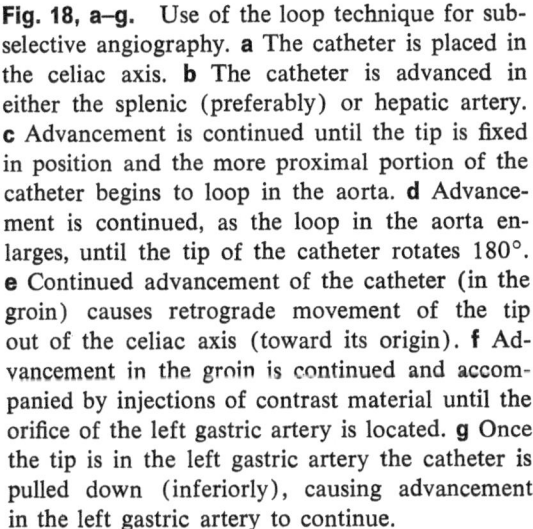

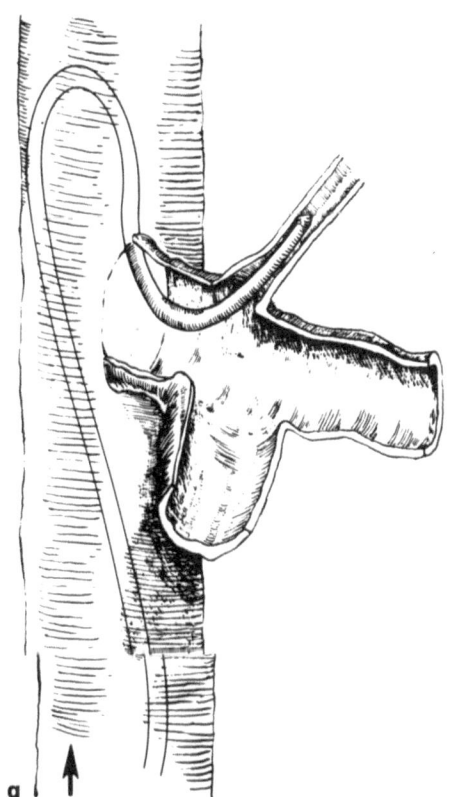

Fig. 18, a–g. Use of the loop technique for subselective angiography. **a** The catheter is placed in the celiac axis. **b** The catheter is advanced in either the splenic (preferably) or hepatic artery. **c** Advancement is continued until the tip is fixed in position and the more proximal portion of the catheter begins to loop in the aorta. **d** Advancement is continued, as the loop in the aorta enlarges, until the tip of the catheter rotates 180°. **e** Continued advancement of the catheter (in the groin) causes retrograde movement of the tip out of the celiac axis (toward its origin). **f** Advancement in the groin is continued and accompanied by injections of contrast material until the orifice of the left gastric artery is located. **g** Once the tip is in the left gastric artery the catheter is pulled down (inferiorly), causing advancement in the left gastric artery to continue.

sels supplying the pancreas and upper abdominal viscera may increase diagnostic yield, and superselective catheterization of the bleeding vessels is necessary prior to therapeutic transcatheter embolization. This section will describe techniques for superselective catheterization of the more commonly studied vessels. A commercially available group of preshaped catheters is demonstrated in Fig. 19. In practice, however, most selective and subselective work may be performed with a standard cobra shape, loop technique, or deflector system, alone or in combination.

The Left Gastric Artery. The left gastric artery is one of the vessels in which superselective catheterization may be essential. Diagnosis of Mallory-Weiss syndrome with active bleeding is often impossible without subselective left gastric injection. Treatment of bleeding in the distribution of the left gastric artery is better facilitated with selective catheterization.

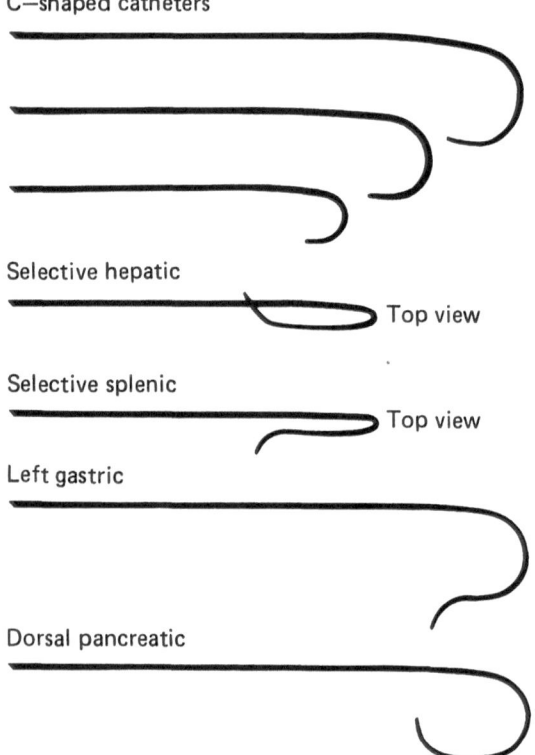

C—shaped catheters

Selective hepatic
Top view

Selective splenic
Top view

Left gastric

Dorsal pancreatic

Fig. 19. Preshaped selective and superselective catheters. Courtesy of Cook Incorporated

The Loop Technique. This technique has been successful in an estimated 85–90% of cases in our experience and has the advantage of avoiding catheter changes, since it is done with the standard cobra catheter. The original technique described by Waltman et al., in which polyethylene catheters and preshaping were necessary, has been modified (see "the Loop Technique in Visceral Angiography").

The "Left Gastric Artery Catheter." This is a preshaped catheter, a 6.3 F with the tip directed at an angle of 180° to the conventional cobra catheter.

Two important maneuvers are necessary: (1) reconstitution of the catheter curve in the aorta and (2) advancement into the celiac axis and the left gastric artery.

1) Reconstitution of the catheter curve. After the catheter is placed in the abdominal aorta it is in the "open" position (Fig. 20). A tip deflector is then passed to the distal end of the catheter without exiting from the tip. Maximum deflection is applied to the tip, which will convert the catheter into a C configuration. With the tip deflected, the catheter is hooked on an aortic branch, i.e., the renal, superior mesenteric, or celiac artery, so that the tip is fixed; the deflector is then released and removed from the catheter. The curve is now reconstituted to its original shape, the tip having a torque factor that causes it to be directed away from the secondary curve.

Other methods may be used to accomplish the same purpose, but with somewhat more difficulty. Occasionally the tip can be manipulated to the contralateral common iliac artery, although this is unlikely because in the open position the catheter behaves like a straight catheter.

The curve can also be reconstituted by using the brachiocephalic vessels; this is accomplished by advancing the catheter after the tip has hooked the orifice of one of the arch vessels. In a tall patient, however, this catheter may be too short to reach the arch.

2) Advancement into the celiac axis and the left gastric artery. After the catheter curve is reconstituted (Fig. 21) all motions are reversed: To advance into the celiac axis the catheter must be pulled back at the groin. To

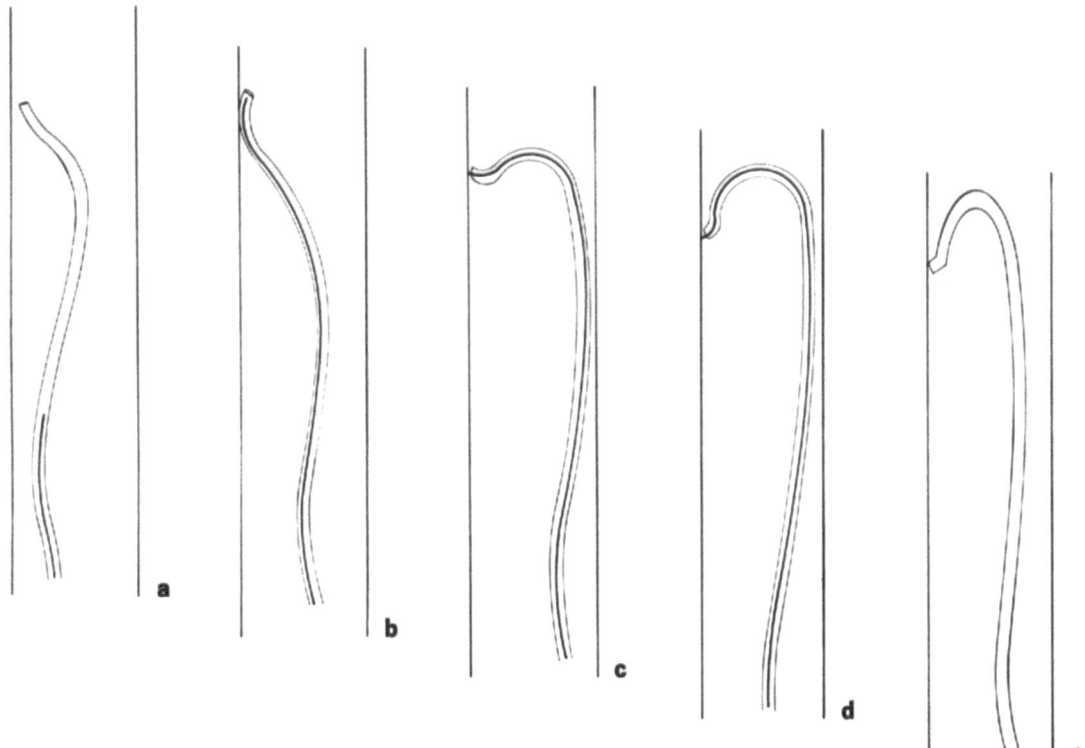

Fig. 20, a–e. Reconstitution of the left gastric artery catheter. **a** After introduction of the catheter into the abdominal aorta the tip is pointing cephalad. **b** A deflector wire is advanced to the tip of the catheter. **c** Deflection is applied. **d** Then complete downward deflection of the tip is accomplished. The catheter is hooked on a vascular orifice. **e** The deflector wire is removed, successfully reconstituting the curve of the left gastric artery catheter.

exit from the celiac axis without losing the curve, the catheter must be advanced at the groin. Once the left gastric artery catheter has been placed in as far as its secondary curve, catheterization of the celiac axis is much simpler than with a conventional catheter because of the downward direction of the tip and because the origin of the left gastric artery is within 1–2 cm of its orifice.

If withdrawal of the catheter at the groin is continued the tip of the catheter will proceed cephalad; and further withdrawal will result in the catheter's "popping" into the orifice of the left gastric artery. An attempt may be made to advance the catheter over a floppy wire, although we have found this to be difficult; it is, in fact, the major disadvantage of this catheter, that is, one may not be able to advance the catheter farther into the left gastric artery if necessary. If the origin of the left gastric

artery is farther from the orifice of the celiac artery than the secondary curve of the catheter, this catheter will not work well. In this instance one could use a "sidewinder" catheter, which has an almost identical shape (see following section), with a longer secondary curve.

The Simmons (Sidewinder) Catheter. This catheter (Simmons 1) is part of the femoro-cerebral series but has found application in visceral angiography as well and can be ordered in lengths more suitable for visceral angiography. Its shape is similar to that of the left gastric artery catheter. A distinct advantage is that it approaches the vascular orifice from a cephalad direction. This may be of particular value in patients in whom the celiac axis is directed downward or in patients with partial celiac obstruction (Fig. 22).

The catheter curve must be re-formed, and

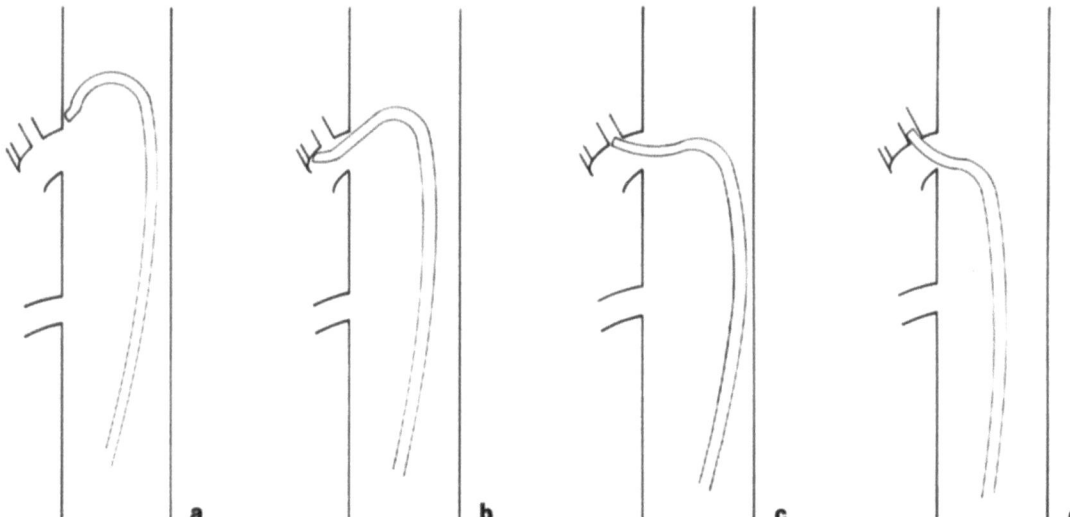

Fig. 21, a–d. Use of the left gastric artery catheter. **a** The catheter is in place in the abdominal aorta (after reconstitution of the curve). **b** In cannulation of the celiac artery orifice the tip will generally pass the orifice of the left gastric artery. Pulling back on the catheter (downward) causes the tip to move along the superior aspect of the celiac axis. **c** Catheter tip is in the orifice. **d** Continued downward movement results in more secure placement in the orifice of the left gastric artery. (*Note:* Continued downward movement will result in retrograde movement of the catheter tip from the left gastric artery and celiac axis into the aorta.)

this may be done quite easily by using the arch vessels. It is of considerable use in selective catheterization of the splenic-hepatic and left gastric arteries as well as of a right hepatic artery originating from the superior mesenteric artery.

The sidewinder 2 has a much larger curve and is somewhat more cumbersome to manipulate; however, it may be of special value for placing the tip far out in the splenic or hepatic artery in a caudally directed celiac axis.

Right Hepatic from Superior Mesenteric Artery

Reshaped Hepatic Catheter. This catheter has a reversed tip, which, when anterior, is directed toward the liver. Reconstitution of the curve is identical to that of the left gastric artery catheter (see above). Once the tip of the catheter is in the superior mesenteric (or celiac) artery it is pulled downward, which will advance the tip distally.

Loop Technique. The catheter is advanced deep into the superior mesenteric artery until the tip will not advance any farther. Continuous advancement in the groin will lead to loop formation, which will cause the direction of the tip to reverse 180°. The catheter is advanced in the groin (which will withdraw the tip from the superior mesenteric artery) with the tip directed toward the right. When the tip reaches the orifice of the right hepatic artery (confirmed by test injection) the catheter is withdrawn in the groin, which will advance the tip into the hepatic artery. The longer the secondary curve, the deeper into the hepatic artery the tip can be passed.

Dorsal Pancreatic Artery. Although originating most often from the splenic artery, occasionally the dorsal pancreatic artery arises from the common hepatic, celiac, or superior mesenteric artery. The standard cobra catheter will work in many instances. A preshaped dorsal pancreatic catheter may also be satisfactory; it has the advantage of having considerable downward torque needed to lodge in the dorsal pancreatic artery. When the artery originates from the superior mesenteric artery the loop technique may be applied.

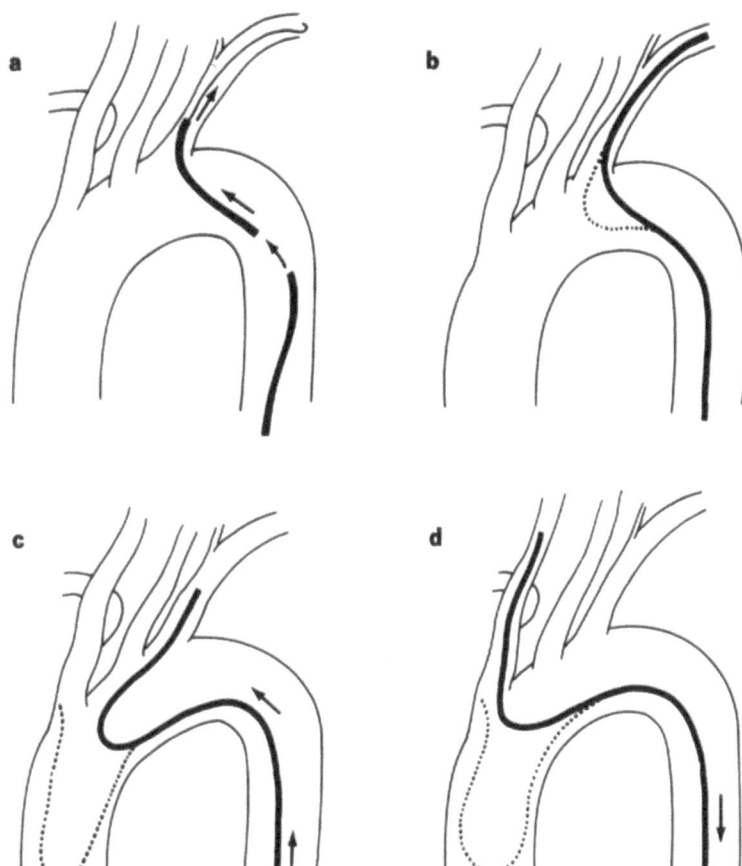

Fig. 22, a–d. Manipulation of the Simmons (sidewinder) catheter in a typical transfemoral approach. **a** Guide wire advanced, catheter to follow. **b** After guidewire is removed to this level, open loop forms as catheter advances. **c** Open loop completely formed as catheter is advanced. **d** Tip ascends to final position as catheter is withdrawn. Simmons CR, Tsao EC, Thompson JR (1973) Angiographic approach to the difficult aortic arch. Am J Roentgenol Rad Ther Nucl Med 119: 605–612

Renal Arteriography

A complete renal arteriogram adequately visualizes the arterial pattern, including the small peripheral ramifications, the nephrographic phase, and the venous phase. Scatter should be reduced by collimation. Aortography may be done prior to selective catheter studies to provide anatomic information in addition to knowledge of pathologic vascular change.

Catheter

Standard cobra catheter, 6.5 F with one side-hole

C-shaped catheter with one side-hole (A single side hole is used to prevent catheter "whip" during injection.)

Injection

4–8 cc/s for 1.5–2 s, depending on size of artery

In cases in which a tumor has been positively identified, "high-dose" injections may be made. Similar flow rates may be used with a volume up to 25–30 cc. This is done predominately to identify the renal vein, and rapid filming in the arterial phase is not necessary.

Film Sequence

10 films: 0.2–0.6 s delay; 2 films/s for 2 s; 1/s for 3 s; 1 film every other second to run out

Total filming, 11–16 s

Technique

After the catheter is placed in the abdominal aorta, maintaining it in a lateral position and searching at the L1–2 level will result in its entry into the renal artery. In catheterization of the renal artery problems arise when there is tortuosity of the aorta or iliac vessels or the origin is aberrant or directed upward. When such tortuosity exists, use of Simmons catheters is helpful.

Aortography will generally localize an aberrant renal artery, although it is not necessary. The other catheterization difficulties may be overcome by use of the loop technique described previously.

Note: When multiple renal arteries are encountered, caution is advised not to inject large amounts of contrast medium, especially into small polar branches.

Coronary Arteriography

The most direct way of evaluating the status of the arterial system is by selective catheteriza-

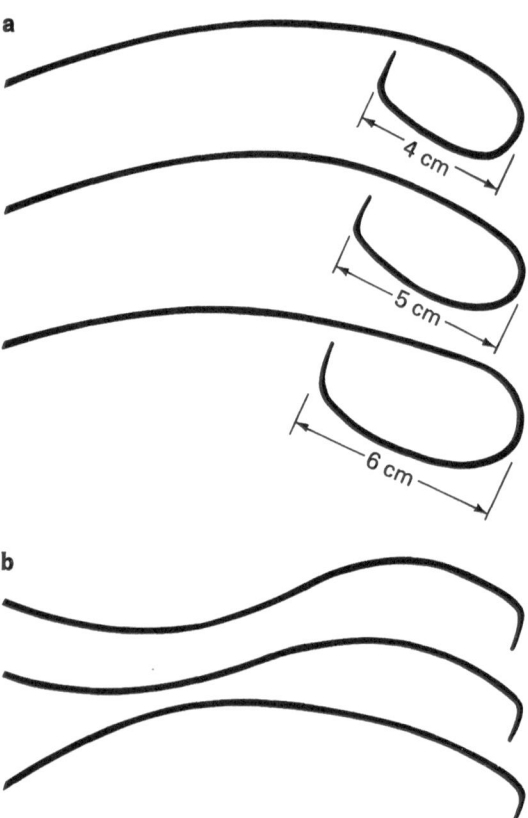

Fig. 23, a and **b.** Coronary artery catheters of the Judkins type. **a** Secondary curves of left coronary artery catheters are of different lengths to accommodate anatomic variations in the aortic arch. **b** Secondary curves of right coronary artery catheters also vary. Courtesy of Cook Incorporated

tion. Although aortic root injections may be of value in some instances, they do not provide the anatomic detail of selective angiography. At present, two major systems of catheterization are in use: Sones technique via right brachial artery cutdown, and the percutaneous transfemoral technique using catheters designed by Judkins or Amplatz. For radiologists skilled in the use of the transfemoral approach, the percutaneous technique offers an extension of those employed in other areas of angiography. The majority of cardiologists performing coronary arteriography use the Sones technique. At our institution coronary angiography is performed by cardiologists and radiologists, both of whom employ the Judkins technique. Familiarity with the Sones technique is worthwhile since occasionally access from the femoral arteries is impossible because of atherosclerotic disease at those sites.

Regardless who performs coronary arteriography, filming, positioning, and interpretation should be supervised by a radiologist.

The Judkins Technique

Left Coronary Artery. The catheter, usually requiring an introducer because of the nontapered tip, is introduced via the standard transfemoral approach. It should be maneuvered into the ascending aorta over the guide, which will maintain the catheter in an open position. Secondary curves of these catheters are of different lengths—4–6 cm—to accommodate anatomic variations in the arch (Fig. 23a).

The patient is turned to a 20°–30° right posterior oblique position, which unfolds the arch in the AP projection. The catheter is then slowly advanced until it drops into the orifice of the coronary artery (Fig. 24). This is done under constant pressure monitoring so that any occluding phenomenon will be immediately noticed. The secondary curve of the catheter in the open position provides sufficient pressure on the tip to maintain it in the orifice.

Since the catheter is designed to almost fall into the ostium of the coronary artery it may be placed in a similar maneuver with the patient in the right anterior oblique position. The characteristic give of the catheter as it drops into the orifice of the coronary artery may be

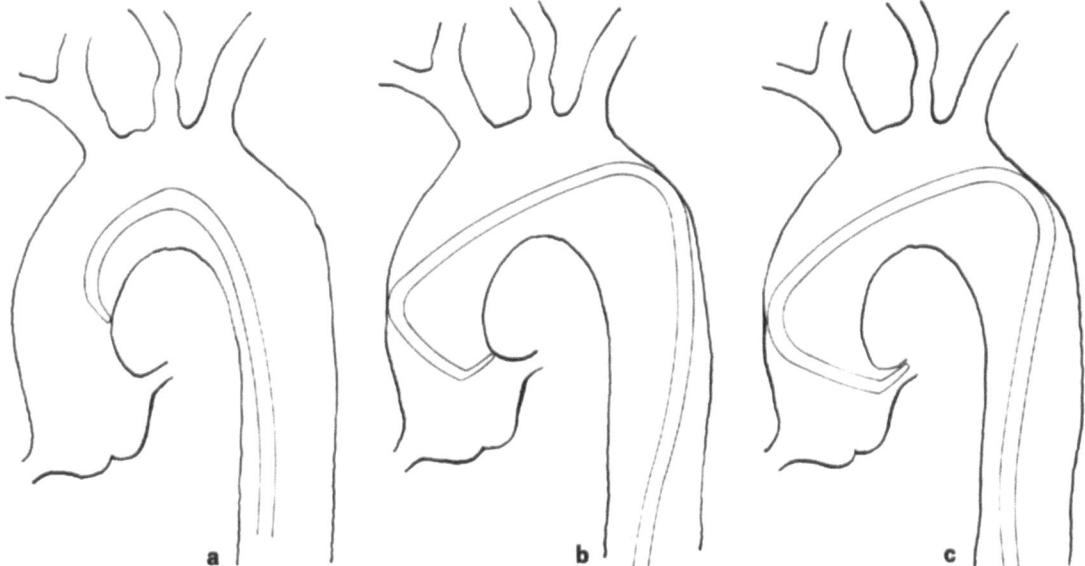

Fig. 24, a–c. Use of left coronary catheter (the Judkins' technique). **a** The catheter is passed in to arch of aorta. **b, c** Continuous advancement results in cannulation of the arterial orifice. From Baltaxe HA, Amplatz K, Levin DC (1976) Coronary angiography. Courtesy of Charles C. Thomas, Publishers, Springfield, Illinois

noted in the left posterior oblique position as well, but this position is less desirable than the right posterior oblique.

Right Coronary Artery. The Judkins right coronary artery catheter is manufactured in three shapes, the main variation being in the secondary curve (Fig. 23b). The catheter is advanced around the arch to a point just above the sinus of Valsalva (Fig. 25). It is rotated

180° and will generally drop into the orifice of the right coronary artery in the same fashion as described previously for the left. Occasionally catheterization of the right coronary artery does require some technical finesse. At first the same maneuver should be repeated at various levels, starting from the sinus of Valsalva and progressing distally along the arch. When the patient is in the 20°–30° right posterior oblique position the ostium generally originates from

Fig. 25, a and **b.** Use of right coronary catheter (the Judkins technique). **a** The catheter is passed into arch of aorta (*dotted* lines) and rotated clockwise. **b** Rotation causes catheter tip to face anteriorly; the catheter is then advanced into the right coronary artery orifice. From Baltaxe HA, Amplatz K, Levin DC (1976) Coronary angiography. Courtesy of Charles C. Thomas, Publishers, Springfield, Illinois

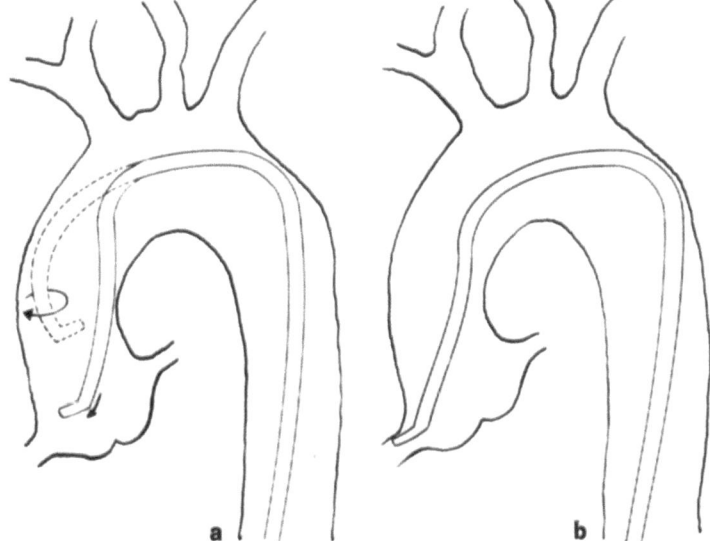

a position tangential to the arch. This is therefore the optimal position to attempt catheterization of the right coronary artery. If this is unsuccessful, consideration might be given to changing to a coronary artery catheter whose shape is not based on arch configuration.

The possibility that the orifice may be occluded should also be taken into account; if the left coronary artery has not been studied this may precede another attempt to catheterize the right coronary artery. If extensive collateral flow is demonstrated to the proximal area of the right coronary artery inability to catheterize this vessel may be due to proximal occlusion. This may be confirmed by arch aortography. Another maneuver that is often effective is to maintain the catheter tip against the anterior wall of the aorta and proceed in an upward motion (cephalad) to the orifice of the coronary artery.

Injection

5–8 cc Renografin-76 by hand injection (tailored to the individual arterial flow and degree of disease visualized at fluoroscopy)

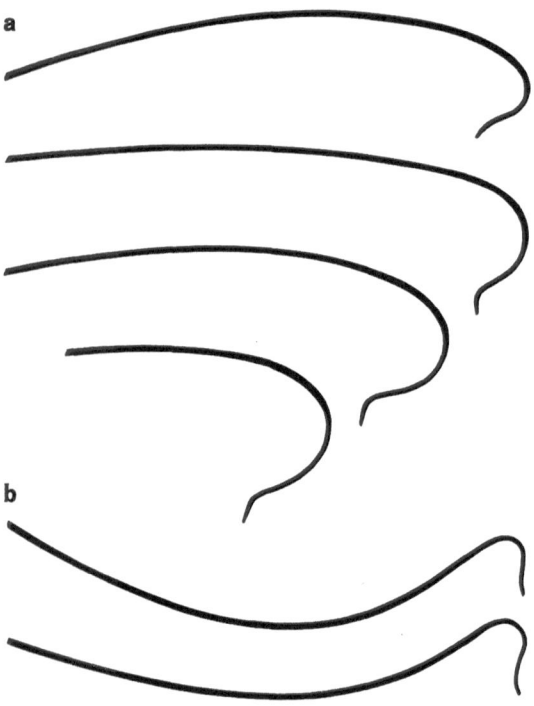

Fig. 26, a and **b.** Coronary artery catheters of the Amplatz type. **a** Left coronary artery catheters; **b** right coronary artery catheters. Courtesy of Cook Incorporated

Filming

Cineangiography
Serial cut films
Photospots

Preferences have been cited for various types of filming for coronary arteriography. Most prefer cineangiography, which provides dynamic visualization of the coronary artery, but with a substantial radiation dose to the patient. With modern focal spots and film-screen combinations, serial cut films or photospots may be obtained that provide high detail and, to an experienced observer, dynamic information. These may be obtained at a rate of 3–6 films/s on most modern spot-film devices and up to 12/s on some newer equipment.

Film Sequence

3–4 films/s for 3 s; 1/s for 2 s
Alternatively, 3–4 films/s for 4–5 s

The Amplatz Technique

Left Coronary Artery. Four catheters designed by Amplatz for use in the left coronary artery are illustrated in Fig. 26a. Choice depends on the individual anatomy of the ascending aorta. This may be predicted with some success from preliminary chest x-rays studies. In general, size 3 is optimal in most males and size 2 in females. This can be evaluated further after the catheter is in place and attempts have been made to catheterize the coronary artery.

The catheter is advanced toward the aortic root so that its J-shaped portion is placed against the aortic valve (Fig. 27). After the ostium has been entered, slight withdrawal of the catheter will cause further advancement into the left main coronary artery. This should be done under fluoroscopic control, with small test injections, and there should be awareness of the catheter's distance within the left main coronary artery. The primary curve of the catheter is designed with a countercurve to prevent wedging into the coronary artery and thus obstruction.

Catheterization of the left coronary artery

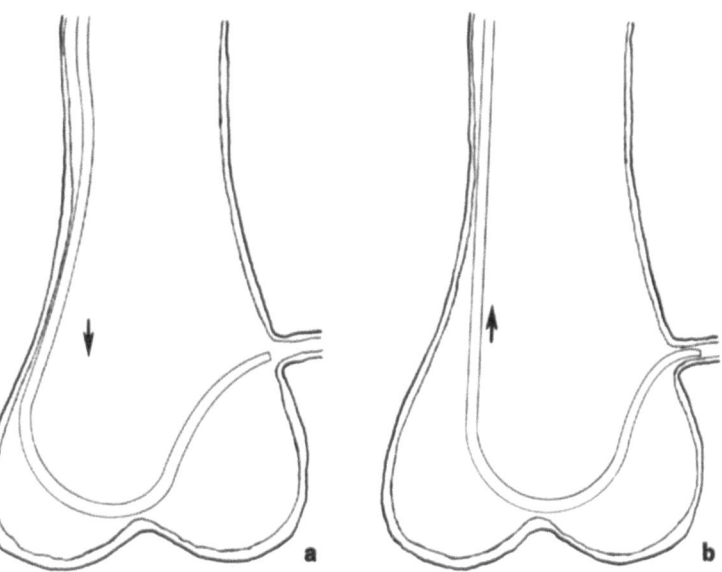

Fig. 27, a and **b.** Use of the Amplatz coronary catheters. **a** The catheter is passed to the root of the aorta and positioned close to the orifice of the coronary artery. **b** Slow retraction of the catheter results in advancement of the catheter tip into the orifice. After Baltaxe HA, Amplatz K, Levin DC (1976) Coronary angiography. Courtesy of Charles C. Thomas, Publishers, Springfield, Illinois

with the Amplatz catheter is more dependent on the catheter–aortic arch configuration than with the Judkins catheter, and catheter change may be helpful. In addition, some rotation of the catheter along the posterior wall of the aorta in the posterior oblique projection may help in successful catheterization.

Right Coronary Artery. The catheters used for the right coronary artery are similar in shape to those for the left coronary artery, but the secondary curve is somewhat smaller (Fig. 26b). The smaller curve is generally satisfactory for most patients, however. The main feature is a reverse curve in the tertiary portion to force the catheter away from the posterior wall. Baltaxe et al. recommended use of fluoroscopy with the patient in the supine position and with the catheter tip pointing directly anteriorly for catheterization of the right coronary artery.

The Sones Technique

In this technique, catheterization of either the left or right coronary artery is performed via a right brachial artery cutdown through which a catheter is placed in the ascending aorta. Under fluoroscopic control the catheter is passed to the root of the aorta. The patient is turned into the left anterior oblique position.

Right Coronary Artery. The ostium of the right coronary artery may be entered directly from a right brachial approach, but care must be taken to prevent occlusion of the vessel by the catheter. Constant monitoring should detect occlusion of the vessel with damping of pressure.

Left Coronary Artery. The left coronary artery is occasionally more difficult to catheterize than the right. The same catheter is utilized. A J shape similar to that of the Amplatz catheter must be formed in the aortic sinus and the catheter manipulated so that the tip is directed cephalad until the coronary ostium is entered.

Bronchial Arteriography

Selective catheterization of the bronchial arteries may be of value in assessing neoplastic disease, benign or malignant, and inflammatory disease. However, in past years the bronchial arteries were one of the areas least often evaluated by selective arteriography. Newer reports point out the value of selective bronchial arteriography and transcatheter embolization in therapy of massive hemoptysis, which may provide the impetus for increased use of selective bronchial arteriography.

Anatomy

Cauldwell et al., after examination of 150 cadavers, defined nine variations in the origin of the bronchial arteries. Figure 28 demonstrates the four most prominent anatomic variations. In 74% of dissections the right and left arose independently; the remainder originated from the common trunk.

On the right, 89% of bronchial arteries arose in a common trunk with the intercostal artery, the great majority from the first intercostal branch of the aorta and the remainder from the second branch. On the left, 70% originated separately from the aorta.

Catheter

Left coronary artery catheter with reverse J shape

Right coronary artery catheter

Several catheters has been described that are effective for selective bronchial catheterization. A catheter with reverse J shape may be effective, for example, the Amplatz left coronary catheter. Also effective is a right coronary catheter of the Judkins type. It is important that the catheter have good torque control and no side-holes.

Injection

Hand injection of 5–8 cc or mechanical injection at low flow rates

Preliminary check of the flow rate under fluoroscopic control to ascertain that catheter will not recoil during filming.

Contrast medium: 76% iodine

Film Sequence

Carried to 10–15 s with allotment for subtraction

For example, 8 films: 2 films/s for 3 s; 1/s to run out

Position

AP or oblique projections, depending on area of interest

Parathyroid Arteriography

A thyroid scan must be obtained *prior* to this procedure.

We presently perform parathyroid angiography primarily for postoperative patients in whom the adenoma is not localized, or in whom symptoms recur. The study is generally done in conjunction with parathyroid venography and subselective venous sampling. Magnification arteriography and subtraction are important adjuncts.

Anatomy

The examiner should have complete knowledge of the anticipated anatomy and anatomic variants prior to performing the procedure. In general, the parathyroid glands receive arterial supply from both thyrocervical trunks (inferior thyroid arteries). It has been shown, however, that some supply does come from the superior thyroid artery.

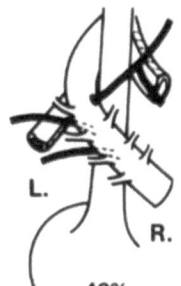 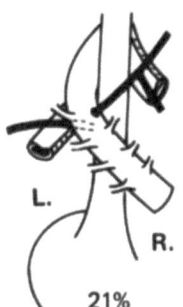 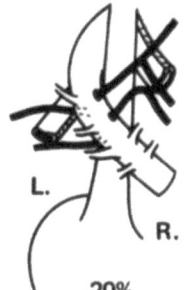 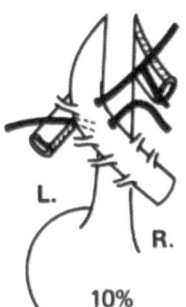

40%　　　21%　　　20%　　　10%

Fig. 28. The most common variations in origin of bronchial arteries. Newton TH, Preger L (1965) Selective bronchial arteriography. Radiology 84: 1043–1051

Purpose

In general, to *localize* an adenoma whose presence is already confirmed by clinical data (This concept is generally valid for most endocrine radiography).

To subselectively inject each of the main branches supplying the parathyroid glands

To study both superior thyroid arteries and the internal mammary arteries if pathologic changes not demonstrated after study of both thyrocervical trunks (Since parathyroid adenomas may be multiple, a complete study may include this entire group of vessels.)

Approach

Usually transfemoral arterial approach

Axillary approach (generally involves bilateral axillary arterial punctures, in which morbidity is increased, and catheterization of the superior thyroid arteries is more difficult)

Catheter

Standard femorocerebral no. 1 or right coronary, depending on arch anatomy

Injection

Superselective injection of thyrocervical trunk and superior thyroid artery: hand injection of 5–10 cc; 5–10 cc at 2–5 cc/s

This should be evaluated under fluoroscopic control prior to filming to avoid excessive reflux into the subclavian or carotid arteries.

Internal mammary artery: 10–15 cc at similar injection rates

Film Sequence

In general, 0.4–0.7 s delay to allow first film to be blank for subtraction
2 films/s for 3 s; 1/s to run out
Filming to 10–12 s

Position

Neck vessels: AP; posterior oblique to ipsilateral side
Mediastinum: Posterior oblique to ipsilateral side

Neuroangiography

Vascular neuroradiology was originally performed by percutaneous puncture in the neck of the appropriate carotid or vertebral artery. It utilized a "minitechnology" developed in an attempt to make these procedures effective, safe, and relatively painless. The direct vertebral injection method soon was replaced by brachial injection. The direct carotid approach is still employed, but in most institutions the femoral approach to the cerebral arteries is preferred.

Occasionally the femorocerebral approach cannot be used, for example when (1) a femoral pulse cannot be palpated; (2) there has been previous femoral-iliac arterial surgery; (3) there is severe aortic-iliac disease that precludes passage of a catheter cephalad; (4) the necessary great vessels cannot be successfully catheterized. In my experience these occur very infrequently, and the femorocerebral approach can be used in all but a few patients.

We find the femoral approach superior for the following reasons:

1) Versatility. It is routine to be able to selectively catheterize and examine all of the intracranial vessels in one study by the femoral route, an impossibility with neck or arm injection and the overwhelming drawback of these older techniques.

2) Ease of femoral artery puncture. Although under usual circumstances puncture of the carotid or brachial artery is relatively easy, puncture of the femoral artery is much easier.

3) Avoidance of patient opposition to neck punctures. Even in the most skilled hands, needle puncture of the neck is often very unpleasant. A large hematoma in the neck may compromise the air column.

Preprocedure Considerations

The appropriate study is determined by consultation between the radiologist and the patient's physician. It is important that this decision be arrived at by mutual agreement; neither the clinician nor the radiologist should arbitrarily defer to the other in selection of the procedure or in its execution.

The procedure is carefully explained to the patient, and consent is obtained and witnessed. Use of premedication is optional. An intravenous infusion is started to allow easy access to the veins and to permit administration of additional sedatives if necessary. Constant electrocardiographic monitoring is utilized.

Femorocerebral Angiography

Technique for Femoral Puncture. See "Femoral Artery" in the section, "The Puncture."

Catheter Irrigation. We use a constant saline drip (heparin is not used) during femorocerebral angiography. This is done by connecting a catheter to a plastic bag of saline surrounded by a pressure cuff. The cuff is inflated to 300 mm Hg, and a reducer is used to permit 1 drop/s to flow into the catheter. This drip continues throughout the procedure. When the pressure injector is used the drip is hooked up through a stopcock, and the stopcock is turned to the injector position just before filming of the series of roentgenograms. It is returned to the drip position as soon as filming is completed.

Some prefer a closed, but not constant infusion, system for flushing to eliminate the possibility of an air embolus. Intermittent flushing may also be used.

"Headhunting" Catheter Technique. A femorocerebral 1 catheter may be routinely used as a starting point in younger patients, but a Simmons 2, 3, or 4 is preferred in patients over 40 years of age. This allows quick catheterization of all vessels without need to change catheters.

Femorocerebral Catheter. The catheter is passed to the top of the aortic arch and is pointed upward, pulled back, and then advanced as the tip enters the innominate artery. Distal to the innominate artery the origin of the carotid is seen with a "puff" of contrast material, and the catheter tip is directed into the right common carotid artery. Slight rotation may be necessary to place the tip more cephalad prior to entry into the carotid artery.

At this point a small amount of contrast agent is injected, and the carotid bifurcation is visualized in order to exclude the presence of a gross abnormality at this level. In most cases the catheter is then advanced only 1 cm into the internal carotid artery because of the possibility of spasm if it is advanced any higher.

To catheterize the left common carotid artery the catheter is advanced into the aortic arch to the distal ascending aorta. The catheter is then withdrawn slowly while the tip is gently pointed cephalad in a manner similar to the technique described in the preceding paragraph for the innominate artery. The catheter will generally proceed into the innominate artery, which may be used as a point for accurate anatomic localization. If the catheter is kept in this configuration, and gentle withdrawal at the groin continued, the catheter will then pass into the orifice of the left carotid artery. It may then be advanced into the left internal carotid artery after the bifurcation is checked fluoroscopically.

The left vertebral artery is larger than or equal in size to the right vertebral artery in more than 70% of patients. Therefore catheterization of the left vertebral artery is usually attempted first. In approximately 10% of patients the left vertebral artery is either too small for catheterization, or it arises directly from the aortic arch, in which case a right-sided study is necessary.

The left subclavian artery is often the easiest of the three great vessels to catheterize. Catheterization may be accomplished by adapting the technique described for the left common carotid artery or by direct passage of the catheter from the lower part of the thoracic aorta. The size of the left vertebral artery should be ascertained prior to selective passage of the catheter into it. If the artery is small the catheter should be withdrawn and the right vetebral artery should be entered via the right subclavian artery. If the left vetebral artery as visualized from the left subclavian artery is normal in size, continuous advancement will cause the catheter to pass into the subclavian artery. A small test injection should be made immediately on entry into the vertebral artery to be sure there is free flow.

Occasionally if both vertebral arteries appear extremely small, the left vetebral artery may arise anomalously directly from the aorta. The catheter is positioned between the left carotid and the left subclavian arteries, at which point the orifice of the left vertebral is usually visualized. Selective vertebral angiography may be performed from this level, or occasionally arch aortography may be necessary for further documentation of the anatomy.

Use of Guide Wires in Femorocerebral Arteriography. The Teflon-coated adjustable wire is a desirable adjunct to femorocerebral arteriography. The catheter tip will frequently enter a vessel, but further pushing on the catheter in the groin merely results in its buckling and failure to continue into the artery. In this case a floppy wire technique is used.

In this technique the wire, with 4 cm of flop, is passed through the catheter into the artery (the catheter itself cannot be advanced over a floppy wire). After the stiff part of the wire has gone beyond the catheter the catheter will then follow the wire up the artery. An alternative is the "push-pull" technique, in which the wire is advanced into the artery, and the catheter is then pushed forward with the left hand while the wire is drawn out of the catheter with the right.

Simmons Catheters. Formerly Shepherd's crook or femorocerebral 4 catheter was used in a tortuous elongated arch in which left carotid catheterization presented a particularly difficult problem. This catheter had two disadvantages: the occasional difficulty in reforming the primary loop in the patient, especially a patient in whom the aortic arch was not dilated, and inability to pass the catheter farther into the artery after the proper vessel had been "hooked." Therefore we now use a Simmons type (sometimes called a sidewinder type) of catheter in an older patient with an elongated arch and tortuous origin of the great vessels.

Since the shape of the catheter is lost in introducing it over the guide wire, the hook must be re-formed prior to use. The easiest vessel to use for this purpose is the left subclavian, which these catheters enter easily when semistraight. The catheter is advanced out the sub-

clavian artery until the curve begins to re-form and the catheter backs out of the vessel. In patients with relatively nondilated and smooth arches a wire may be necessary to stiffen the catheter just proximal to the large U of the hook. With the wire at this point the catheter almost always backs out with its proper shape.

Advancement of the properly shaped catheter into the ascending aorta allows easy entry into the innominate artery by means of a simple withdrawal technique at the groin. The catheter may enter the carotid artery directly or, failing that, a guide wire may have to be used to place the catheter in that vessel.

Catheterization of the left carotid artery is achieved by the same withdrawal technique. In order to bypass the innominate artery the catheter must be rotated at the groin to allow the tip to just slip by the orifice, following which the tip is again directed cephalad and the orifice of the carotid artery carefully searched. Counterclockwise rotation usually enables the tip to avoid the orifice of the innominate artery, but whichever rotation performs best in the individual patient is satisfactory. A stiffening wire is often necessary to permit advancement of the catheter further into the left carotid artery, but in some extreme cases, only the most proximal part of the vessel can be engaged and a proximal injection must be made.

The easiest vessel to engage is the left subclavian, from which the left vertebral artery is usually easily entered with the upward hooking tip of the catheter. Care must be taken not to plug the artery with the catheter; an extremely tortuous origin of the vertebral artery often allows only very proximal placement of the catheter.

Delivery of Contrast Medium. There is no place for constant-pressure injectors in modern neuroradiology. Therefore an injector that has a feedback mechanism to allow injection of a constant volume is used in all studies. For the carotid artery a flow rate is chosen that is "sufficient to fill." In this technique an approximate flow rate is chosen, and a test injection is made at this rate under fluoroscopic control. If the contrast substance "backs down" the flow rate chosen is too high and is reduced proportionately. Conversely, if the contrast material is diluted and passes up the artery a proportionately faster flow is used. With a proper rate of injection the contrast medium passes neither up nor down the carotid artery under the fluoroscope (obviously, and in fact, the contrast agent is constantly being infused and constantly moving up the artery).

Usually a flow rate of 7–9 cc/s for a total of 12 cc is chosen for the common carotid artery and about 6 cc/s for the internal carotid artery for a total of 10 cc. For vertebral artery injection the flow rate is approximately 5–7 cc/s for a total of 8 cc. Diatrizoate 60% is the contrast material used.

Pullout. After the serial films have been completed the catheter is withdrawn to the external iliac artery, about 4 cm above the puncture site in the groin. A small needle is placed over the skin puncture site to identify it. The catheter is then connected to the power injector, a test injection is made at a rate of 5 cc/s for a total of 5 cc, and the puncture site is examined fluoroscopically. If any abnormality is detected a formal pullout angiogram is obtained with the multiple-film changer. If the femoral puncture site appears normal a pullout angiogram may be obtained with a spot-film device and $2\times$ magnification.

Following this the operator firmly presses the superficial femoral artery just *distal* to the puncture site. An assistant connects a syringe to the catheter and aspirates blood while the catheter is slowly withdrawn from the femoral artery. Two heart beats are allowed to force blood from the femoral artery onto the skin before the operator's hand is transferred above the puncture site to compress the femoral artery. The assistant "squirts" the withdrawn blood onto the draping sheets to see if any clots have been withdrawn. Clots are visible in about 25% of cases.

The assistant then feels the posterior tibial or dorsal pulse in the foot. When the assistant claims to feel the pulse the operator asks the assistant to count the pulse aloud. When the presence of a foot pulse is confirmed the operator knows the femoral artery is being compressed only to the point of reduction of flow and not to the point of obliteration. Compres-

sion is then applied for 5–10 minutes, by which time the artery will usually stop bleeding and seal itself.

The patient is instructed not to flex the leg for 24 hours and to walk "stiff legged" for the same period. I do not like leaving a patient in bed for 24 hours after a femoral puncture and have been very happy with the stiff-leg technique. It has also been accepted much better by patients and floor nurses.

I do not put any kind of bandage over the femoral puncture site so that any bleeding can be immediately detected. If a patient is unconscious or uncooperative an actual visual check is kept of the puncture site for at least 2 hours after the study.

All patients, especially male patients, are warned of the physiologic diuresis that will occur with the use of a large amount of contrast material.

Direct Carotid Arteriography

The neck is put in hyperextension by placing a large bag under the shoulders as a wedge. The neck from the mandible to the clavicles is prepared and draped. The carotid artery is felt in the neck (the most prominent pulsation occurs at the carotid bifurcation at approximately C-4. A point halfway between the prominent pulsation and the clavicle is selected for skin puncture; this allows needle entrance into the common carotid artery below the bifurcation. A skin wheal is made, and the needle for anesthesia is passed medial to the carotid artery and lateral to the trachea, all the way posteriorly to the anterior longitudinal ligament. A relatively large amount (8 cc) of procaine is injected at this area to elevate and move the common carotid artery laterally. A small amount of anesthestic can be placed laterally, although I frequently omit this part of the anesthesia. The carotid artery is forked between the index and middle fingers of the left hand, and the artery pierced through and through with a needle (Potts-Cournand) in the right hand. The needle is turned so the bevel is down and slowly withdrawn from the artery until pulsation is obtained. Then, as the needle is depressed and advanced, its tip comes to lie in the center of the lumen of the artery.

The study can be done at this time. A Potts handle or "brace" may be required to depress the needle so the bevel will not lie against the posterior carotid wall.

Alternatively the needle may be advanced over a short wire or a fine no. 7 sheath catheter placed over the wire and into the carotid artery. This results in a much smoother procedure, but a disadvantage is that the catheter occasionally goes into the external carotid artery, and repositioning it into the internal carotid artery can be a nuisance. Flow rates are similar to those used under similar circumstances for femorocerebral catheterization. Following the study the catheter or needle is withdrawn, and pressure is applied to the carotid until bleeding stops.

Note:

1) Needle or catheter position should be double-checked under fluoroscopy or by low-volume Polaroid radiography prior to filming.
2) Presence of the needle or catheter in the external carotid artery may be suspected when pain following test injection contrast of the medium is in the distribution of the external carotid artery branches (i.e., occipital or temporal discomfort).
3) Often, blanching will occur over the roof of the orbit following saline injection in the internal carotid artery (superior ophthalmic branches).

Brachial Arteriography

In the brachial technique the arm is placed in external rotation and the brachial artery palpated in the medial antecubital fossa. After induction of anesthesia a Potts needle is placed in the brachial artery and carefully threaded up it. The position of the needle is carefully checked by fluoroscopy; the presence of muscular branches affirms that the needle is in the lumen and not subintimal.

The contrast medium is injected rapidly (approximately 25 cc/s for a total of 40 cc). It refluxes up the brachial artery and will often fill the left vertebral. An overwhelming advantage of this artery technique is that it is very safe; however, it will afford satisfactory posterior fossa angiography in only two-thirds of patients. In spite of the large amount of contrast agent in the brachial artery, complications involving the hand are virtually nonexistent.

5 Venous Examinations

Venography of the Lower Extremity

Purpose

The aim of lower extremity venography is to opacify as completely as possible the deep venous structures from the ankle to and including the inferior vena cava. Opacification of the superficial veins is generally of little clinical value and may obscure the deep structures. Venography has been found to be useful in the following clinical situations.

Thrombophlebitis: To evaluate the deep venous structures for presence or absence of thrombi

Varicose veins: To evaluate patency of the deep veins and to demonstrate incompetent perforators

Swollen leg and venous stasis syndromes: To assess the structure and function of the deep venous system

Venous anomaly: To determine the size and extent of blood supply to the lesion.

Patient Positioning

Supine on a tilting fluoroscopy table (television preferred) with head of the table elevated to 45°.

Patient's entire weight is supported by leg not being studied to fully relax the muscles on the side being examined. A telephone book may be placed under the contralateral foot for this purpose.

Injection

120 cc 45% meglumine

Dilute low-sodium contrast material causes less discomfort. Mix 60% contrast: 2 parts contrast to 1 part normal saline.

Film Sequence

The following films were taken on a 14 × 17. Films are properly collimated.

1) Frontal view of the calf to include knee
2) Lateral view of calf to include knee
3) Lateral view of leg centered on knee
4) Frontal view of leg centered on knee
5) Frontal view of thigh
6) Lateral view of thigh
7) Frontal view of pelvis to include lower inferior vena cava
8) Frontal view of lower abdomen to include inferior vena cava as completely as possible

Technique

A tourniquet is placed tightly above the ankle. A superficial vein on the dorsum of the foot is selected for cannulation. The most distal vein suitable should be chosen. A 21-gauge butterfly needle is used, taped securely in place. Edema may often be massaged away to reveal a vein for cannulation. Rarely, a cutdown may be necessary.

Slow infusion of normal saline is begun and the needle position checked for any signs of infiltration or swelling. If either is present, the needle must be repositioned. (Skin sloughing has occurred following subcutaneous injection of high volumes of contrast medium.)

A second tourniquet is placed tightly above the ankle, the patient positioned, and the tube and film readied for exposure.

Inject contrast steadily over 60–90 seconds. After 60 cc of contrast material is injected, and during injection of the second 60 cc, the first seven films listed are taken in order as quickly as possible. Gentle yet firm pressure is applied over the femoral vein in the groin and the table is returned to the horizontal position; the leg being studied is elevated, the groin pressure released and the final film exposed. This maneuver will often enhance visualization of the pelvic venous structures and inferior vena cava. Tourniquets are now removed.

If evaluation of the "muscle pump" is required, the patient should remain in the 45° head-up position and forcefully flex the sole of the foot ten times against the examiner's hand. After this exercise, a second set of frontal and lateral calf films is exposed.

If the venous structures are satisfactorily visualized, the leg is elevated slightly and the remainder of the normal saline is infused and the needle removed. If an area was poorly filled or an abnormality suspected, a repeat injection with spot filming can often provide valuable additional information. Occasionally, the iliofemoral veins and inferior vena cava will not be adequately visualized and a direct femoral vein puncture may be necessary for complete evaluation.

A final film of the abdomen to evaluate the kidneys, ureters, and bladder may be taken if indicated.

Pitfalls

The venous anatomy of the lower extremity is quite variable, and pathologic changes often appear as obstruction. The examiner must always keep in mind that normal veins may not fill on any one injection, and if this is suspected to be the case a repeat injection with fluoroscopic monitoring will often resolve the question. The head of the table can be further elevated and the calf gently palpated during reinjection in an attempt to fill the veins in ques-

tion. Occasionally, there is a relative paucity of deep venous structures in normal individuals. Sometimes the needle may have to be repositioned more distally on the dorsum of the foot to better fill the deep veins.

Flow of unopacified blood into an opacified column of blood will produce a "filling defect." This usually has a characteristic configuration, generally not identical in the multiple views routinely obtained. A repeat injection will almost always allow differentiation between a true thrombus and a flow defect.

Superior Venacavography

The diagnosis of the superior vena cava syndrome is often apparent clinically and may be graphically demonstrated by superior venacavography. More subtle defects may only be seen radiographically.

Purpose

To obtain visualization of the superior vena cava and major thoracic venous tributaries

Injection

Simultaneous hand injection into both basilic venous systems of 30–50 cc diatrizoate meglumine and diatrizoate sodium (Renografin-60)

Unilateral injection may be used, but flow defects may occur that may provide difficulty in interpretation.

Film Sequence

10 films generally. Filming to 10 s at 1/s
In severe superior obstruction of vena cava: to 20 s to adequately visualize all collateral pathways

Film rate may be tailored to the rate of injection and suspected degree of obstruction.

Technique

Technique is based on the prevalent venous anatomy in which a large medial *basilic* (Fig. 29) venous system drains into the axillary and subclavian veins, and a considerably smaller *cephalic* system courses laterally and superiorly. An 18-gauge short intracath is placed in each basilic venous system. (Smaller-gauge needles may be used with subsequent sacrifice in flow rate through the smaller caliber.)

Inferior Venacavography

Purpose

To demonstrate morphologic detail of inferior vena cava and collateral pathways in cases of obstruction

Injection

20–25 cc/s diatrizoate meglumine and diatrizoate sodium (Renografin-76) over 2 s.

Y connector from the injector in simultaneous injections (In this case, flow rates must be doubled on the selector.)

Film Sequence

Filming in AP and lateral projections advisable 0.5-s delay 3 films/s for 2 s; 1/s for 3 s

When caval obstruction is suspected, longer filming should be considered for optimal visualization of collateral pathways.

Technique

This procedure may be performed with bilateral needle puncture, with Teflon sheaths, and simultaneous injection, or with single-catheter injection. The latter may be subject to some pitfalls in diagnosis, especially as a result of flow from the opposite lower extremity.

Renal Venography

Purpose

To adequately visualize the main renal vein, intrarenal tributaries, and communications with the capsular and retroperitoneal venous system

Catheters

Standard cobra with side-hole alternatively, C-shaped or J-shaped

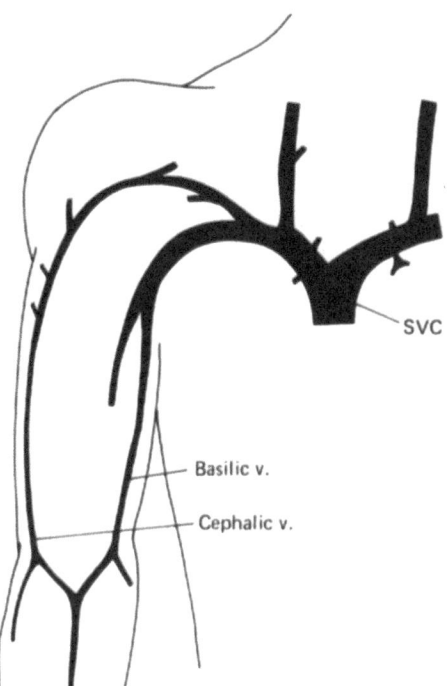

Fig. 29. Anatomic basis for needle localization. The medial basilic venous system represents a direct communication with the larger axillary-subclavian-innominate venous system (*SVC*), whereas the lateral cephalic venous system represents a smaller more circuitous route.

Injection

7–10 cc/s for total of 15–20 cc (If epinephrine is not used flow rates should be considerably higher.)

Film Sequence

2–3 films/s for the time of injection (2 s); 1/s for approximately 5–7 s

Technique

Venous puncture and catheter placement are as described for inferior venacavography. The renal veins are catheterized relatively easily by moving the catheter superiorly with the tip pointing laterally toward the desired renal vein. Once the catheter has entered the renal vein it should be advanced to reduce reflux into the vena cava. (Because of the length of the left renal vein the catheter should be placed proximal to the gonadal vein.) The renal vein may be studied at this point; however, adequate filling of the small veins will not be obtained because of the extremely high rate of flow through the renal *arteries*. To alleviate this problem, small amounts of epinephrine (5–8 μg) should be administered selectively into the renal artery on the side to be studied. Contrast medium may be injected into the renal vein 10–20 s after the intra*arterial* injection of epinephrine.

Pulmonary Angiography Transfemoral Approach

Purpose

To adequately visualize the main pulmonary artery and all peripheral branches (This is best obtained by selective right and left pulmonary arteriography.)

Equipment

Side-hole-only catheter (NIH, Eppendorf)
Entry sheath (Desilets)
Specially designed pigtail catheter (Grollman) with L curve (Fig. 30) (An advantage of this catheter is that it can be placed by the Seldinger technique; a disadvantage may be less than optimal for subselective pulmonary arterial injections.)
Deflector (may be of considerable help in subselective catheterization)

Injection

Main pulmonary artery: 25–30 cc/s for 1.8–2.0 s

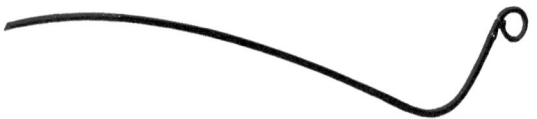

Fig. 30. Pulmonary artery pigtail catheter, Grollman type. The L shape facilitates passage through the tricuspid valve and pulmonary outflow tract. Courtesy of Cook Incorporated

Selective pulmonary artery: 15–25 cc/s for 1.5 s
Right atrium: 20–25 cc/s for 2.5–3 s

Right atrial injections for the purpose of determining presence of pulmonary emboli should be avoided if possible because of lower diagnostic accuracy. Magnification in association with subselective pulmonary branch injections has been shown to be extremely helpful in demonstrating pulmonary emboli and should be employed in the segments questioned by lung scan if not seen by selective studies (the "scan-directed arteriogram").

Film Sequence

Main pulmonary artery: 0.5–0.8 s delay
Selective pulmonary artery: 0.5–0.8 s delay
3 films/s for 3 s; 1/s for 3 s

Technique

ECG monitoring is required.

Pulmonary arterial pressure should be monitored by the standard manifold technique. If this is not available a water manometer may be used, the readings being converted mathematically to millimeters of mercury.

A gentle curve should be shaped in the distal 5–7 cm of the sheath. The catheter is placed into the right atrium. Subsequent advancement and counterclockwise rotation will lead the catheter tip into the main pulmonary outflow tract.

Note: Normal pressures: right atrium, 3 mm Hg; right ventricle, 27/4 mm Hg; pulmonary artery, 13 mm Hg (mean), 20/4 mm Hg.

If there is pulmonary hypertension, the possibility of acute failure should be weighed against the clinical necessity of obtaining the arteriogram, although only rarely will the examination be impossible. If pulmonary pressure is greater than 70–80 mm Hg, termination of the study should be seriously considered, to avoid refractory heart failure.

In patients in whom left bundle-branch block is noted on the ECG, a temporary pacemaker should be placed because complete heart block might be induced by passage of the catheter into the right ventricle.

Adrenal Venography

Anatomy

Figure 31 depicts the anatomy of the supra-renal veins.

Purpose

To delineate the contour of the adrenal gland
To evaluate adrenal masses, including hyper-plasia, adenoma, and pheochromcytoma

Equipment

Red Kifa catheter (left vein), C-shaped or 30° angle (right vein)
Polyethylene cobra catheter without side-holes (left and right veins)
Left coronary artery catheter (right vein)
Simmons's sidewinder 2 catheter (left and right veins)
Preshaped adrenal catheter (left and right veins)

The function of the Simmons sidewinder type of catheter (Fig. 32) is identical to that of the preshaped adrenal catheter (Fig. 33). Each catheter is quite useful in both adrenal veins (Fig. 33). The sidewinder 2 is pre-ferred because the secondary curve is long enough to permit the tip to enter the adrenal vein, even when it is proximal (deep) to the renal vein. It may be readily used to cathe-terize the right adrenal vein directly.

Injection

Hand injections preferred in both venous sys-tems, started at a slow rate and then in-creased if left adrenal vein is large
Mechanical injection 2–3 cc/s for 3–4 s

Extreme care must be taken because both adrenal glands may be easily ruptured during injection of the contrast agent. Considerable pain may be associated with both injections even without rupture. This should be evaluated individually by test injection under fluoro-scopic control. In sufficient pressure during in-jection will result in abnormal findings.

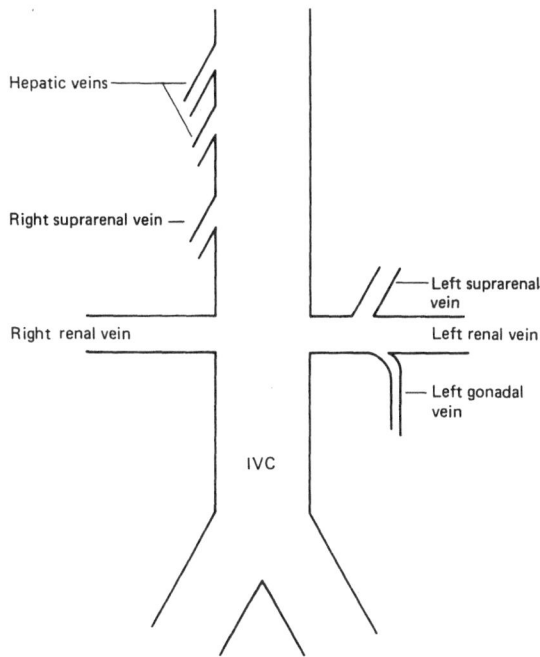

Fig. 31. Suprarenal venous anatomy. *IVC*, in-ferior vena cava.

Film Sequence

10 films generally
Hand injection over 2–3 s: 2 films/s; 1/s or 1 every other second for approximately 10 s (This is extremely variable, depending on the individual flow and individual injection rates.)

If subtraction is considered, a single film should be exposed prior to the injection.

Left Suprarenal Vein

Technique

Three techniques may be used to catheterize the left suprarenal vein. In the first, a red Kifa catheter may be shaped, on the basis of the local anatomy, as shown in Fig. 34. If this is done the catheter will be of no use in cathe-terizing the right side, and a new catheter must be shaped. With a red Kifa catheter of this design a deflector is used to introduce it into the renal vein. The catheter is then advanced distally and the deflector removed. Simple de-

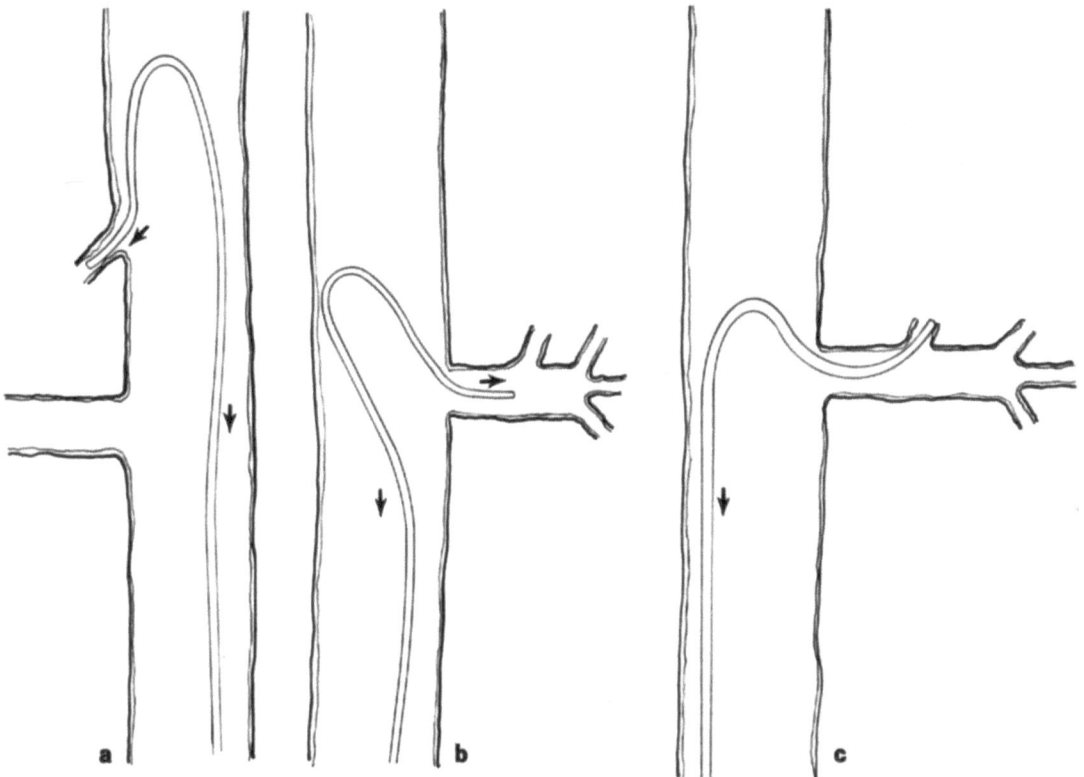

Fig. 32, a–g. A Simmons' shape catheter for suprarenal venography. **a** After reconstitution of the curve, the *right suprarenal vein (arrows)* is catheterized. **b** The *left suprarenal vein* is catheterized by first placing the catheter tip in the left renal vein. Continuous downward movement of the catheter results in advancement of the tip farther into the renal vein. **c** Continuous downward movement directs the tip upward. This motion is continued until the tip "pops" into the orifice. (A guide wire should not be passed into the suprarenal vein but may be used within the catheter to add torque.) **d–g** (*facing page*).   **d** Radiograph demonstrating cobra catheter at the orifice of the left renal vein. **e** The catheter is advanced in the inferior vena cava, while the tip is fixed against the wall of the left renal vein. **f** Advancement of the catheter continues until simultaneous formation of a loop in the inferior vena cava and 180° reversal of the catheter tip. **g** After formation of the loop, further advancement of the catheter in the inferior vena cava results in the catheter tip moving toward the suprarenal vein until cannulation is achieved. Once the tip enters the orifice of the suprarenal vein, movement of the catheter downward from the groin results in advancement of the catheter tip into the suprarenal vein.

traction of the catheter will allow the upward-directed tip to be placed in the suprarenal vein.

This technique is of little value in present-day angiography since it involves catheter shaping and is not applicable to the right suprarenal vein.

In the second method a polyethylene cobra catheter (without side-holes) is used. The tip is placed in the renal vein and advanced into its more peripheral tributaries. At this point the loop technique, described originally by Waltman for left gastric artery catheterization, is employed. The catheter is advanced against fixed resistance at the tip. Subsequently a loop is formed in the inferior vena cava, upon which the tip in the renal vein reverses and is pointed upward. With the catheter in this configuration all movements are reversed, that is, if the catheter is advanced in the groin it moves out of the renal vein toward the inferior vena cava, and if the catheter is retracted in the groin, its tip advances farther into the renal vein (Fig.

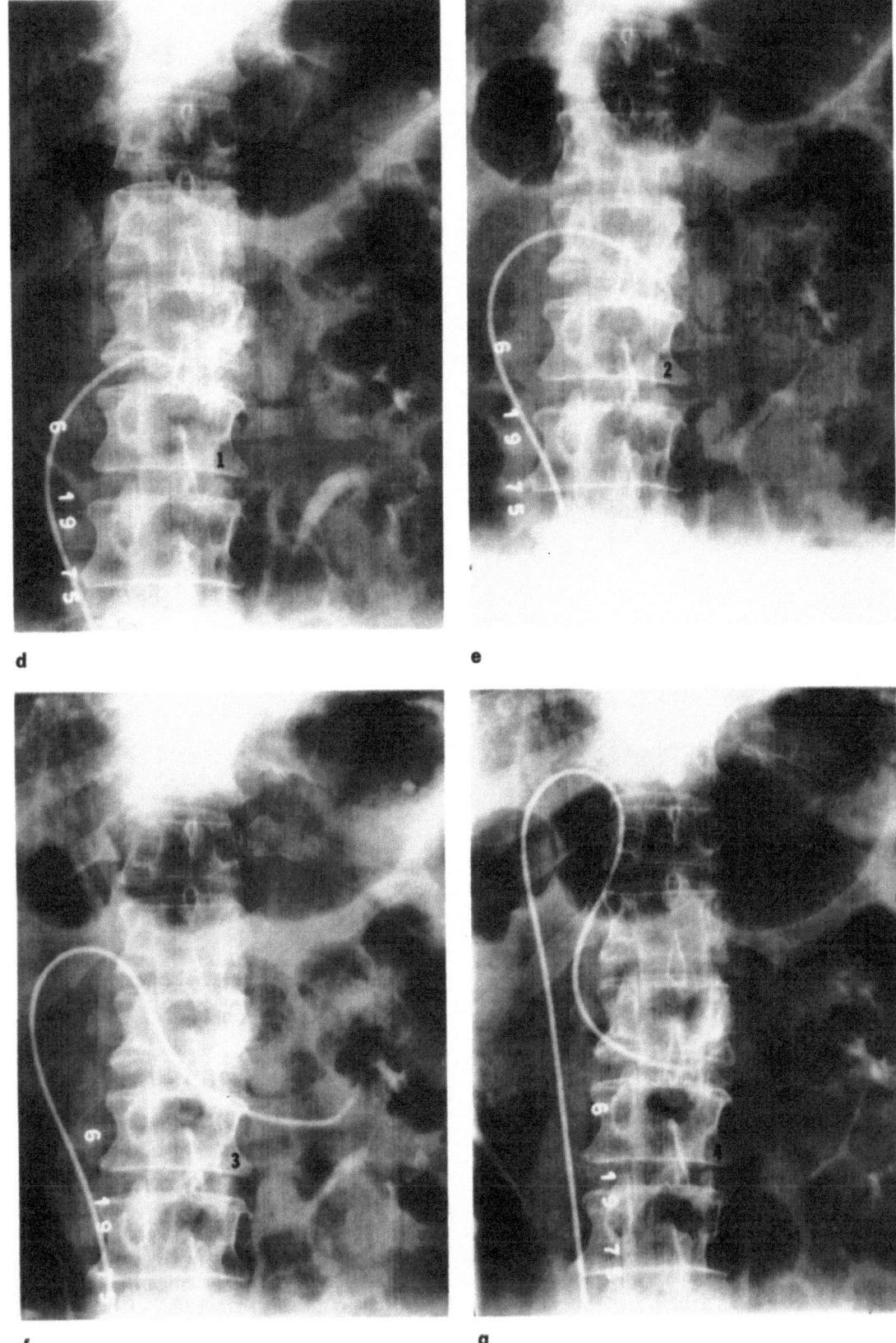

d

e

f

g

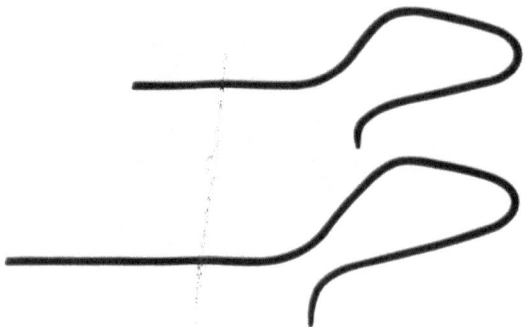

Fig. 33. Preshaped suprarenal catheters. Courtesy of Cook Incorporated

35). The catheter is then manipulated into the suprarenal vein.

A third method employs a Simmons catheter or pre-shaped suprarenal vein catheter. Both have inferiorly directed tips when the catheter curve is reformed in the inferior vena cava.

Right Suprarenal Vein

Technique

If a cobra catheter has been used for catheterization of the left vein then an attempt may be made to use it for the procedure in the right suprarenal vein. The right vein is somewhat more difficult to catheterize because of its origin from the inferior vena cava and its variability in site. In addition, several hepatic veins drain into the inferior vena cava in this region and must be differentiated during the study.

Other catheters reportedly used successfully in catheterization of the right suprarenal vein include a red Kifa catheter with a C-shaped or a 30° angle, a left coronary artery catheter, and a pre-shaped suprarenal catheter. Utmost care must be exercised with the coronary catheter because it is rather stiff and the venous intima is easily traumatized.

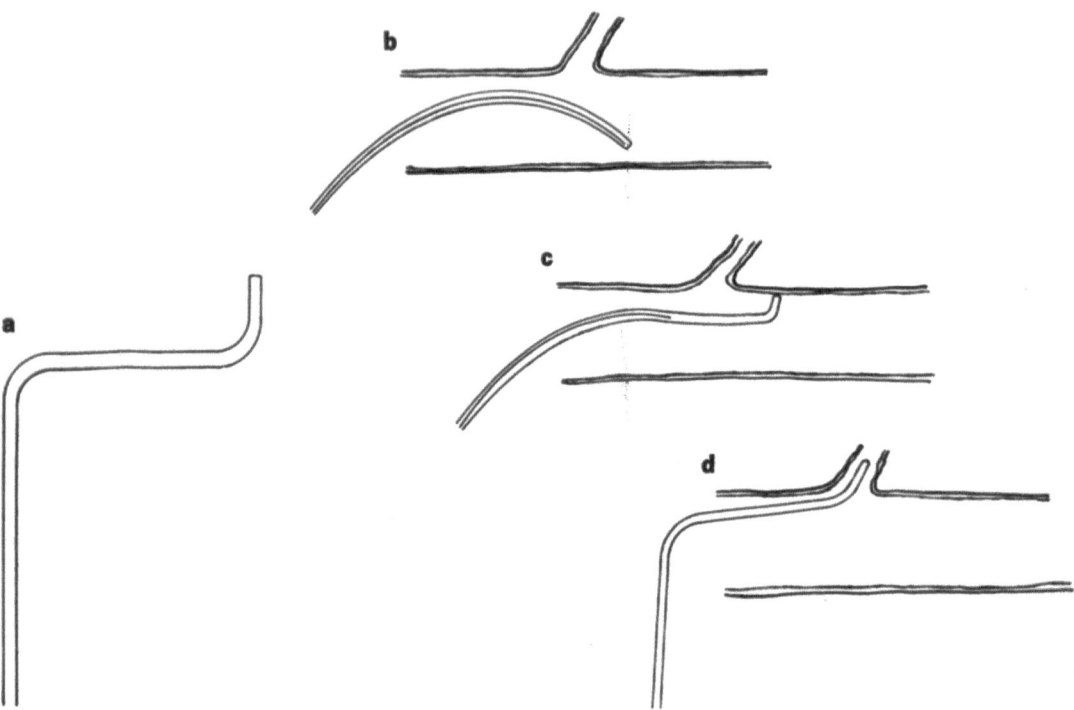

Fig. 34, a–d. Suprarenal venography via catheter shaping in the angiography suite. **a** A catheter is shaped with two right-angle curves, the secondary curve measuring approximately 4 cm in length. **b** After the catheter is placed in the venous system the left renal vein is cannulated with the wire in place in order to eliminate the preshaped curves. **c** The catheter assumes its original shape after the wire is removed. **d** Retrograde movement of the catheter results in cannulation of the adrenal vein.

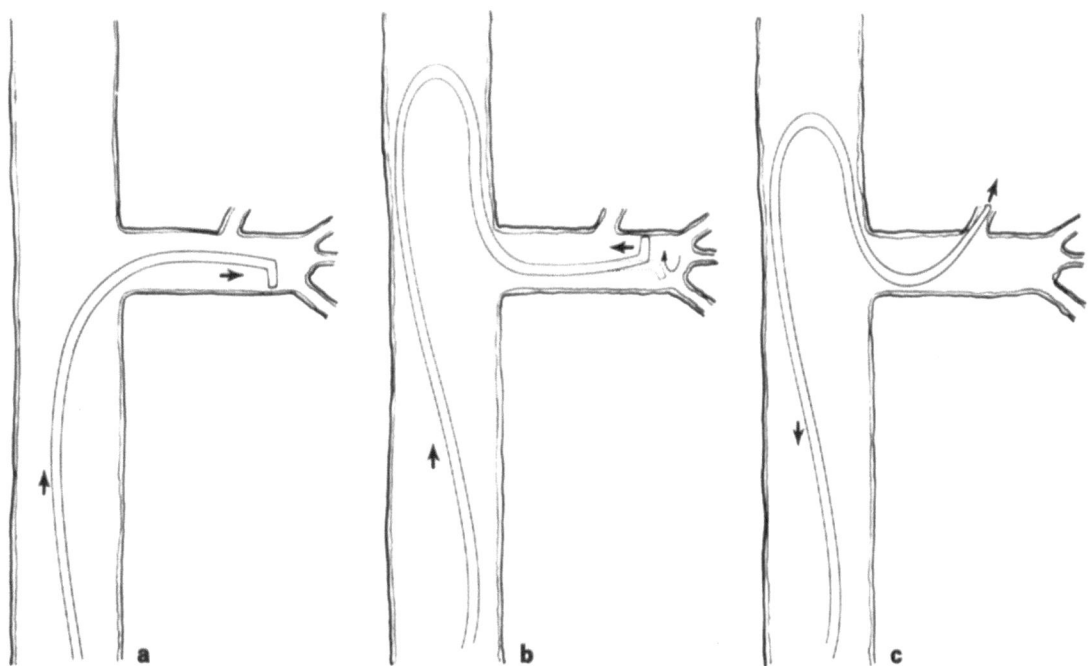

Fig. 35, a–c. The loop technique for supravenal venography. **a** The left renal vein is cannulated. **b** The catheter is advanced until loop forms, resulting in simultaneous reversal of the catheter tip (by 180°). Continuous advancement at the groin will cause the catheter tip to withdraw from the renal vein until the tip reaches the adrenal vein. **c** Once the left suprarenal vein is cannulated retraction in the groin will cause the tip to advance farther in the suprarenal vein.

Thyroid Venography

Venography and venous sampling may be extremely helpful in localizing parathyroid adenoma (Fig. 36).

Purpose

To adequately visualize the entire thyroid venous plexus

To sample blood from the mediastinal veins for parathormone assay in parathyroid abnormality

Catheter

Femorocerebral no. 1 or right coronary

Injection

Generally a total of 8–10 cc over 2–3 s (This will vary according to the size of the veins.)

If the inferior thyroid vein is selectively catheterized, filling of the entire venous system should be attempted; if successful this will obviate the need for further injection of contrast medium.

Film Sequence

In general, 10 films: 0.4–0.7 s delay to allow
    initial film to be blank for subtraction
2 films/s during initial 3 s
Filming to 10–11 s

Technique

Examination of this type should be preceded by adequate study of the venous anatomy and its variations. The transfemoral approach is preferred. Because of the venous anatomy (Fig. 37), catheterization of the inferior thyroid vein, which is generally single, should be attempted first. If this is successful, injection of the contrast agent will generally fill the entire thyroid plexus. In addition to the inferior thyroid veins, both superior thyroid veins (branches of the jugular) should be catheterized and injected.

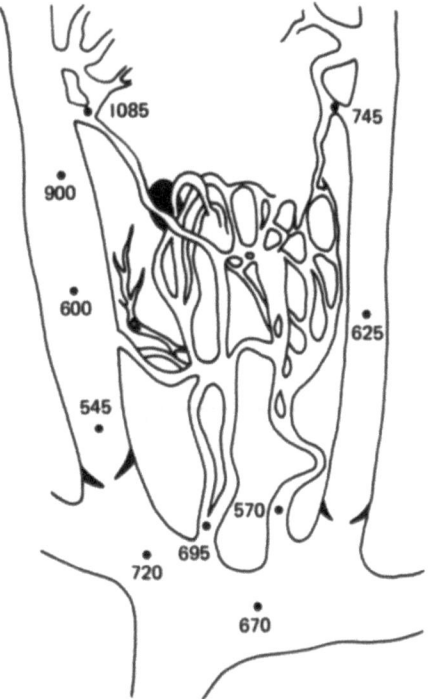

Fig. 36. Subselective thyroid venography to obtain blood for parathormone assay. Measurements of parathormone from various regions of the internal jugular and thyroid veins are shown, in addition to the location of the parathyroid adenoma. The highest elevations were obtained from the right superior thyroid vein, closest to the parathyroid adenoma. Der Maur GAP et al. (1975) Parathyroid venous sampling. Radiol Clin, Biol 44:1–13

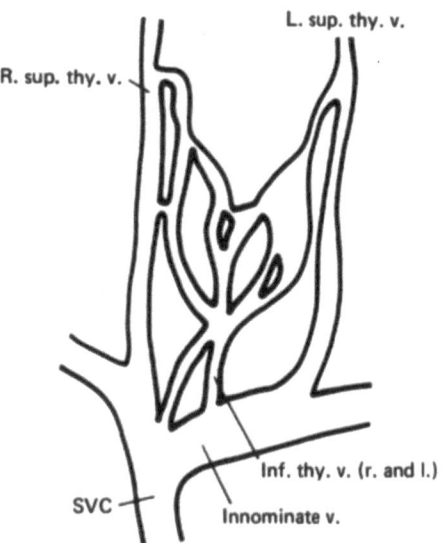

Fig. 37. The pertinent thyroid venous anatomy.

Superselective venous sampling for parathormone has been shown to be quite helpful in locating parathyroid tumors. Cardiac status should be monitored while the catheter is passed through the right atrium.

Azygography

Purpose

To evaluate intrathoracic disorders causing displacement, deformity or obstruction of the azygos vein

To visualize lung neoplasms (? resectability), esophageal carcinoma, metastases to mediastinal lymph nodes

To identify cause of hydrothorax, e.g., thrombosis of the azygos vein

To differentiate mediastinal masses located in the right tracheobronchial angle

To assess status of esophagus after radiation therapy

Transcostal

Equipment

Diatrizoate sodium (Hypaque 50%) no. 18 spinal needle or no. 16 bone marrow (Rosenthal) needle

Plastic tube connector 15 cm long

Injection

Hand injection: 25 cc contrast medium over 6–7 s

Note: Needle is left in place until films are checked.

Film Sequence

Exposure at midinjection
2/s for 10 s

Position

Biplane AP and lateral projections (tip edge of film should include clavicles)

Note: If a second injection of contrast agent is needed more lidocaine should be introduced into the medullary cavity of the rib.

Technique

The patient is permitted nothing by mouth before the procedure. Demerol 100 mg and seconal 100 mg are administered 1 hour before the procedure.

Puncture usually is made in the midaxillary line in the ninth or tenth left rib after preparation of the area. Anesthesia is induced with lidocaine (Xylocaine 1%) down to the periosteum. The needle is introduced obliquely through the soft tissues and then redirected so that the tip can be used to feel the superior and inferior borders of the rib. The needle is placed at an angle of 90° with the outer cortex of the rib. With a rotatory motion the obturator within the needle "bites" the cortex of the rib. The needle is tilted along the axis of the rib with the tip directed posteriorly. The medullary cavity is penetrated, and the needle advanced for 3–5 mm and compressed. *The aspirate should contain bone marrow.*

Note: If there is a bulge of the soft tissues with this injection the needle should be advanced or rotated and then, after the tube is flushed, connected with the plastic connector and a 30-cc syringe containing contrast medium.

Transfemoral

Catheter

Headhunter (femerocerebral 1)

Injection

8–12 cc/s for 20–25 cc diatriazoate meglumine and diatrizoate sodium (Renografin-76)

Film Sequence

Biplane; 2 films/s for 10 s

Technique

The femoral vein is punctured and the catheter placed in the superior vena cava. With the right tracheobronchial angle used as an anatomic landmark, the posterior wall of the superior cava is explored, usually slightly medially. As the orifice of the azygos vein is being sought, a test injection is made to rule out obstruction of the very distal azygos vein. If there is obstruction the catheter is advanced for a few centimeters.

Epidural Venography

Although herniated lumbar disk classically was demonstrated by means of iophendylate (Pantopaque) and more recently, water-soluble contrast myelography, a potentially more sensitive means, epidural venography, has been introduced. Opacification of epidural veins that lie in intimate contact with the posterior margins of the vertebral bodies and intervertebral disks is easily accomplished by transfemoral selective catheterization. As any surgeon who has performed lumbar disk surgery can attest, the veins lying anterior to the caudal sac are the last structures to be traversed prior to excision of herniated disk material. These veins, which cause so much difficulty at the operating table, provide the radiologist with the most sensitive indicator of lumbar disk disease.

The most important technical aspect of this study is to ensure complete filling and opacification of all veins above, below, and at each disk level. If this is not accomplished an accurate diagnosis cannot be made.

Anatomy

Simply the pattern of venous anatomy is fairly constant and consistent although the detailed venous anatomy may vary widely between individuals. The entire caudal sac (and spinal cord at higher levels) is surrounded by a vertebral plexus lying in the epidural space (Fig. 38). The anterior group of veins comprising this plexus, the anterior internal vertebral veins, are of importance in the interpretation of epidural venograms. The epidural venous plexus is connected to veins lying outside the bony spinal canal (ascending lumbar veins and their continuation) by numerous valveless communicating veins, the largest and most constant of which are the superior and inferior pedicular veins. In the AP projection, which is the most commonly used, the vertebral

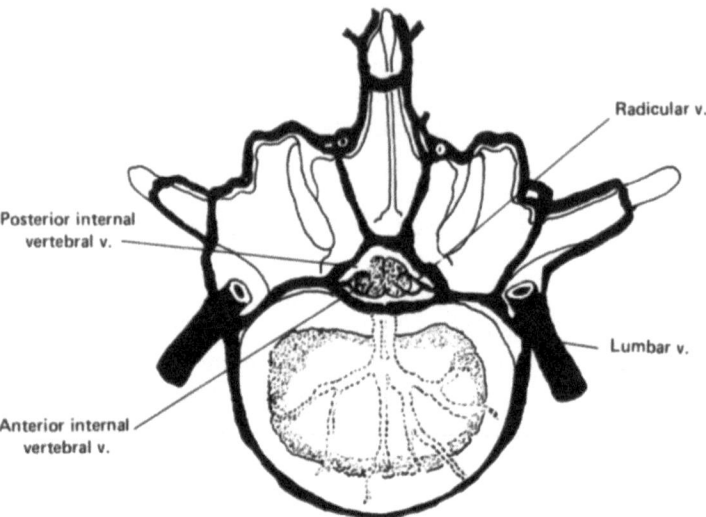

Posterior internal vertebral v.

Anterior internal vertebral v.

Radicular v.

Lumbar v.

Fig. 38. Cross section of the lumbar spine demonstrating the relationship of the epidural veins to the dural sac, vertebral disks, and nerve roots.

venous plexus is seen to form a more or less hexagonal pattern because of the relative narrowing of its transverse diameter at the level of each pedicle pair (Fig. 39).

Since the veins are valveless and interconnecting, opacification of the internal vertebral veins at all levels in the lumbar region is relatively simple by catheterization of one or two veins. The ascending lumbar vein arises from the superior aspect of each common iliac vein at approximately the level of the first sacral foramen. The angle of origin of the left ascending lumbar vein makes catheterization of this vein easier than that of the right. At lower levels there are several sets of cross-connecting presacral veins that arise from branches of each internal iliac vein. A complete study is usually obtained with injection of one or both of these veins.

Purpose

To demonstrate herniation of an intervertebral lumbar disk or the presence of spinal stenosis

Equipment

5 F 50-cm polyethylene catheter
Deflector wire if necessary

Since many of the veins are quite small and fragile, catheterization should be performed with the above-listed catheter. Only a 50-cm catheter is required since the veins are a short distance from the puncture site. The short distance also allows easy control of the soft, floppy catheter. A simple 45° bend at the distal end of the catheter will generally allow selection of all the desired veins. A deflector wire may be used to provide more curvature if necessary.

Injection

2–5 cc/s
20–30 cc total

The venous system is a very slowly flowing, high-capacitance system, and therefore slow injection rates are needed. Higher rates will only cause accentuation of the reflux, which almost always occurs into the iliac veins and inferior vena cava, and are more likely to burst a small vein. The upper limit of the suggested rates has worked well in the ascending lumbar veins while the lower rates applies more to the presacral veins. The total volume of the vertebral plexus is small. The smaller volume limit applies to presacral injection.

Filming

Usually AP projection only
Sometimes lateral views (mandatory for spinal stenosis)
Sometimes oblique views

Although lateral views may be helpful in confirming displacement of a vein they are of

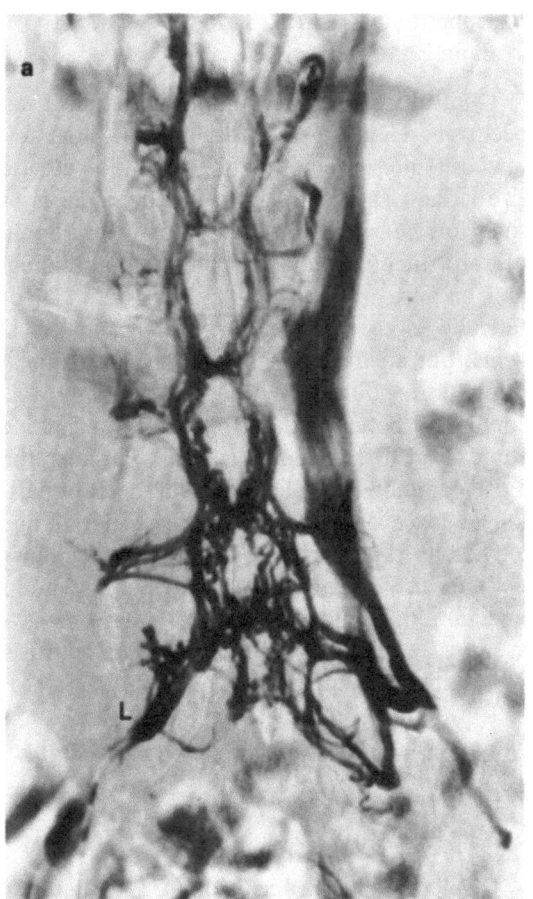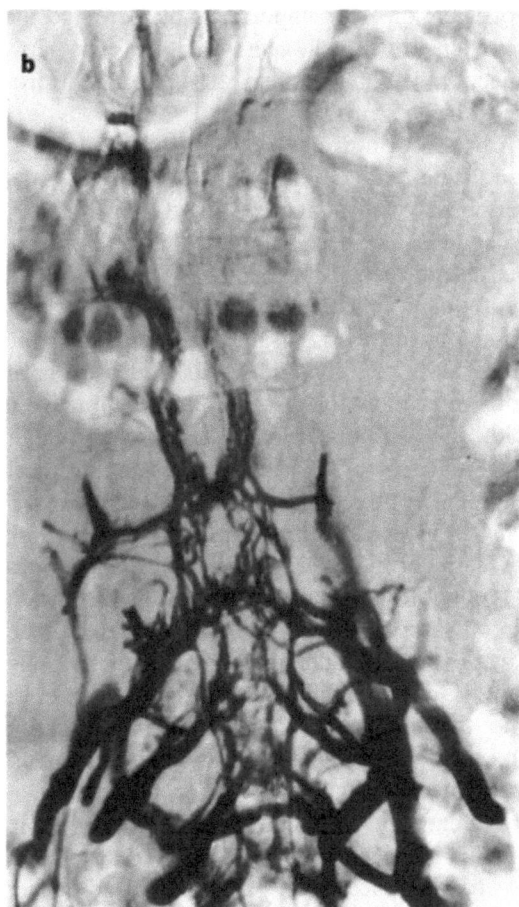

Fig. 39, a and **b.** Lumbar epidural venography. To avoid incomplete venous filling, injection of multiple sites may be necessary. **a** Injection of contrast in the ascending lumbar vein (*L*) demonstrates the normal hexagonal pattern of the epidural venous plexus; however, the L5-S1 interspace is not well demonstrated. **b** Injection of contrast agent in the presacral venous plexus better demonstrates the lower levels.

no use when a vein is completely occluded. Oblique films have been used by some, but in almost all cases, the diagnosis may be made from the frontal films alone.

Film Sequence

1 film/s for 10–12 s

Subtraction films are almost essential since opacification of the vertebral plexus is often faint and obscured by the vertebrae, particularly at the upper levels. A mask prepared as the films are being developed helps to quickly determine if further injections are necessary to completely fill the veins.

Technique

The left femoral vein is chosen because, as noted, the angle of origin of the left ascending lumbar vein makes entry into it easy. After introduction of the catheter into the vein by the standard Seldinger technique, the tip is directed cephalad and the upper surface of the left iliac vein slowly searched by means of small test injections until the ascending lumbar vein is entered. Frequently the major trunk of this vein quickly branches into numerous small twigs, and the catheter should not be introduced too far into the orifice until it is certain that a major trunk continues cephalad. Injection at the orifice will usually give satisfactory opacification. It is important not to wedge the catheter into small veins because even slow injection will burst them and result in retroperitoneal extravasation.

In most individuals, injection of the left ascending lumbar vein will opacify the internal vertebral veins at levels from L4-5 to L2-3. Adequate opacification above this level is rare because of the small capacity of the system and consequent reflux into the major veins. Less common, however, is satisfactory filling of the veins at levels from L5 to S1 because major communications of the ascending lumbar vein with the vertebral plexus begin at a higher level. Therefore it is usually necessary to inject one of the intercommunicating presacral veins. This is most easily accomplished by directing the catheter into the right iliac vein. Sometimes it is possible to "bounce" the downward-directed tip off the right lateral wall of the inferior vena cava. With a gentle nudge the catheter may slide down the wall of the inferior vena cava into the more perpendicular right iliac vein. Once this occurs the tip is automatically forced medially and usually falls into a presacral vein. If the catheter cannot be prevented from rising up the inferior vena cava rather than sliding down it, a deflector wire may be used to deflect the tip more acutely downward so that it can enter the right iliac vein.

Complications

Bleeding
Venous thrombosis
Dislodgment of clots from pelvic veins
Air embolization

Retroperitoneal extravasation of contrast medium

Clinically significant complications have not occurred. Hemostasis is easily controlled following femoral venipuncture since the catheter size is kept small and the venous system is at such low pressure. Venous thrombosis should be rare since catheter manipulation is minimal and because of the small catheter size. Theoretically clots may be dislodged from pelvic veins, but adequate history taking and clinical evaluation should detect patients in whom this could be a potential danger. Careless technique could lead to air embolization. Perhaps the most common complication will be retroperitoneal extravasation of contrast material due to venous rupture from wedging the catheter tip into tiny branches or from too great an injection rate into small veins. These extravasations are mildly painful but usually cause no significant problems.

It would be judicious to defer studies on patients who are receiving anticoagulation therapy.

Interpretation

Displacement or occlusion of the anterior internal vertebral veins is the key to diagnosis. Displacement may, at times, be quite subtle, but since the anterior internal vertebral veins are paired there should be a normal vein for comparison at each level except when there is bilateral occlusion or bilateral lateral displacement by huge herniated disks. Occlusion will be noted at the level of any prior surgical intervention. Interpretation is considered in detail in articles listed in the bibliography.

6 Special Procedures

Musculoskeletal Arthrography

Although arthrography can be performed on any joint into which a needle can be inserted, the majority of arthrograms are of the knee, followed in decreasing order of frequency by arthrograms of the shoulder, hip, ankle, wrist, and elbow. The contrast material used in arthrography is 60% or 76% meglumine diatrizoate or iothalamate. The meglumine salts are preferred as the sodium salts may cause severe pain if extraarticular injections occur.

In single-positive-contrast arthrography, water-soluble contrast material is injected into a joint. Single-positive-contrast arthrography is the method of choice in determining whether ligaments, tendons, or joint capsules are ruptured. Radiopaque loose or foreign bodies within a joint, however, may be obscured by the opaque contrast material.

In double-contrast arthrography, water-soluble contrast material and air are injected into a joint. Double-contrast arthrography is best for evaluation of cartilage because a thin layer of contrast material over the cartilage is outlined by the air within the joint. Air bubbles surrounded by contrast material may occasionally simulate loose bodies.

Negative-contrast arthrography may be used in evaluation of radiopaque loose or foreign bodies within a joint. Negative-contrast arthrography gives poor contrast and poor detail of the internal structures of the joint.

Scout films of the joint should be available and should be reviewed before any injection is made. Strict sterile technique is used throughout the injection procedure. Arthrography should not be performed if there is skin infection near the site of the needle puncture. When the needle enters the joint, any fluid present should be aspirated. If the fluid is cloudy or if infection is suspected, the fluid should be sent to the laboratory for culture and sensitivity studies. Clear serous fluid from a joint usually does not have to be sent to the laboratory if there is no suspicion of infection. If chondrocalcinosis (pseudogout) is present or suspected, the fluid should be sent for evaluation of crystals.

Water soluble contrast material is absorbed fairly rapidly from a joint so that radiographs should be obtained without any delay after the injection. Since filming of the arthrogram may have to be modified in view of the suspected pathologic finding a brief clinical history should be obtained from the patient prior to the injection.

Purpose

To visualize the nonradiopaque internal structures of a joint, including the cartilage, ligaments, and synovium

To determine if loose bodies are present in a joint

To determine if ligaments around a joint are intact or ruptured

To determine if soft-tissue masses around a

joint are cysts or abscesses that communicate with the joint

To confirm that a needle inserted into a joint for aspiration is intraarticular

Equipment

Standard arthrography tray, including: drape with 2 × 2-in. opening in center 20-, 10-, and 2-cc syringes

16-, 18-, 20-, and 22-gauge 1.5-in. disposable needles 25-gauge 0.75-in. needle

4 × 4-in. gauze pads

Forceps

Sterile 30-in. Plastic tubing (Venotube)

Additional needles, if necessary after set is opened

Complications

Allergic reactions

Vasovagal reactions

Infection

Allergic reactions may occur as water-soluble contrast material is absorbed by the synovium and enters the bloodstream. No fatal reactions have been reported after arthrography, and the usual allergic reaction consists only of urticaria. Still, the benefit of the arthrogram has to be weighed against the rare possibility of serious allergic reaction in patients with a history of allergy to water-soluble contrast material.

Vasovagal reactions occasionally occur during or after the injection procedures. These are not allergic reactions. Patients with vasovagal reactions will become diaphoretic, nauseated, dizzy, and may faint if put in the upright position. Hypotension and bradycardia occur. Treatment consists of placing the patient in the Trendelenburg position so that blood will flow to the head. Patients usually recover rapidly so that the filming can continue after brief treatment, Atropine, with an initial dose of 0.4 mg intravenously, can be used to treat a vasovagal reaction; however, this is seldom necessary.

Infection is a potentially very serious complication of arthrography; fortunately it is very rare if a sterile technique is used.

Knee Arthrography

Purpose

To demonstrate tears of medial and lateral menisci

To demonstrate tears of medial collateral ligament

To visualize tears of cruciate ligaments

To evaluate popliteal cysts, pigmented villonodular synovitis, loose bodies, osteochondral fractures, and osteochondritis dissecans

Injuries to the cartilage, ligaments, or joint capsule of the knee can lead to symptoms of pain and limitation of motion, termed internal derangement of the knee. Internal derangement of the knee frequently occurs after athletic injury.

Arthrography is very accurate in the diagnosis of tears of the medical meniscus. Accuracy decreases somewhat in tears of the lateral meniscus; however, most abnormalities of the lateral meniscus can be demonstrated. The degree of accuracy achieved in the diagnosis of meniscus tears will, of course, depend on the technical quality of the arthrograms and on experience in interpreting them.

Tears of the medial collateral ligament can be demonstrated on arthrography within 48 hours of injury. After this, the joint capsule may seal over and become watertight so that the tear cannot be demonstrated.

Equipment

Reciprocating grid, fine-line grid, or lead insert to reduce scatter

Restraining device

20-gauge 1.5 in. disposable needle

High-quality arthrograms by the fluoroscopic spot-film method required a small focal spot measuring 0.3–0.6 mm for the fluoroscopic tube. Arthrograms obtained with the focal spot measuring more than 1 mm will not show as sharp an outline of the menisci as a result of magnification artifact. The usual fluoroscopic tube contains two focal spots, a small and a large. Fluoroscopy is performed with the small focal spot, and when spot films are obtained, usually the machine automatically switches to the large focal spot. Most fluoroscopic machines will have to be modified by installation of a special switch so that spot films can be obtained with a small focal spot.

Scatter may decrease the quality of films made without a grid. A reciprocating grid in the fluoroscopic tower is very useful. A stationary fine-line grid can also be used; it usually does not interfere with interpretation of the arthrogram. Some arthrographers remove the stationary grid and put in its place a lead insert with a cutout the size of the spot film they want to obtain; this also is useful in reducing scatter. Phototiming is generally not used because the field size is usually too small to obtain good results. We use 60–70 kV at 100 mA at 1/20 or 1/15 s. The actual technique used will depend on the size of the patient and the equipment used.

Patient Positioning

Prone
Varus or valgus stress to knee

A restraining device is needed that will allow varus or valgus stress to be applied to the knee. We use the abdominal restraining band that came with the fluoroscopic table. (Fig. 40) One of the hooks was removed, and both pieces of the cloth restraining band were attached to the single hook. The restraining band should be adjustable to the size of the patient.

A restraining device for arthrography is now commercially available.

Film Sequence

6 or 9 exposures on each film

Manual collimation is used so that either six or nine exposures can be made on each film. In order to obtain six exposures on a film, four exposures are obtained on the 4 on 1 setting, which will place an image in each of the four corners, and then two exposures are placed in the center of the film on the 2 on 1 longitudinal-split setting (Fig. 41). In order to obtain nine exposures, there must be manual collimation to a very small field size. Then the 4 on 1 split, longitudinal 2 on 2, the horizontal 2 on 2, and the 1 on 1 settings are exposed

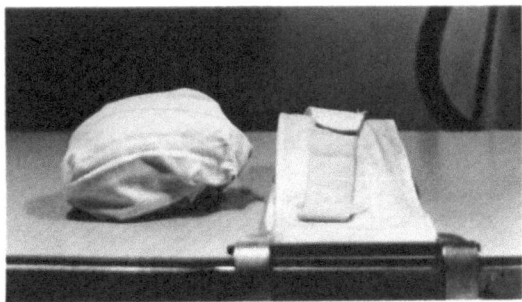

Fig. 40. The sling, which attaches by hooks to the side of the table, was made from the abdominal restraining band that came with the fluoroscopic table. A cushion for underneath the knee was made by wrapping a cloth around gauze rolls. A towel may also be used.

(Fig. 42). We prefer having six exposures on a film so that the field size is somewhat larger, which will allow us to see the position of the femoral condyles.

Technique

The preliminary AP, lateral, skyline, and tunnel views of the knees are reviewed. A short history is obtained from the patient so that the procedure can be modified if necessary. The patient is placed on the fluoroscopic table in the supine position with a small cushion under the popliteal fossa. The injection site, which should be beneath the mid portion of the patella in the space between the patella and femoral condyles (Fig. 43), is shaved, scrubbed with povidone-iodine, and draped.

The needle can be inserted from either the medial or lateral aspect of the knee. An ordinary 20-gauge 1.5-inch disposable needle is used for the injection. The patella is displaced toward the side of the injection as this serves to widen the space between the patella and femoral condyles. The patient is instructed to try to relax the knee, and especially not to tighten the quadriceps muscle as this will decrease the space between the patella and femoral condyles.

A local anesthetic may be used; however, usually we do not find it necessary as there is only minimal pain when the needle goes through the skin. Pain does occur, however, if the needle strikes the bony surfaces of the pa-

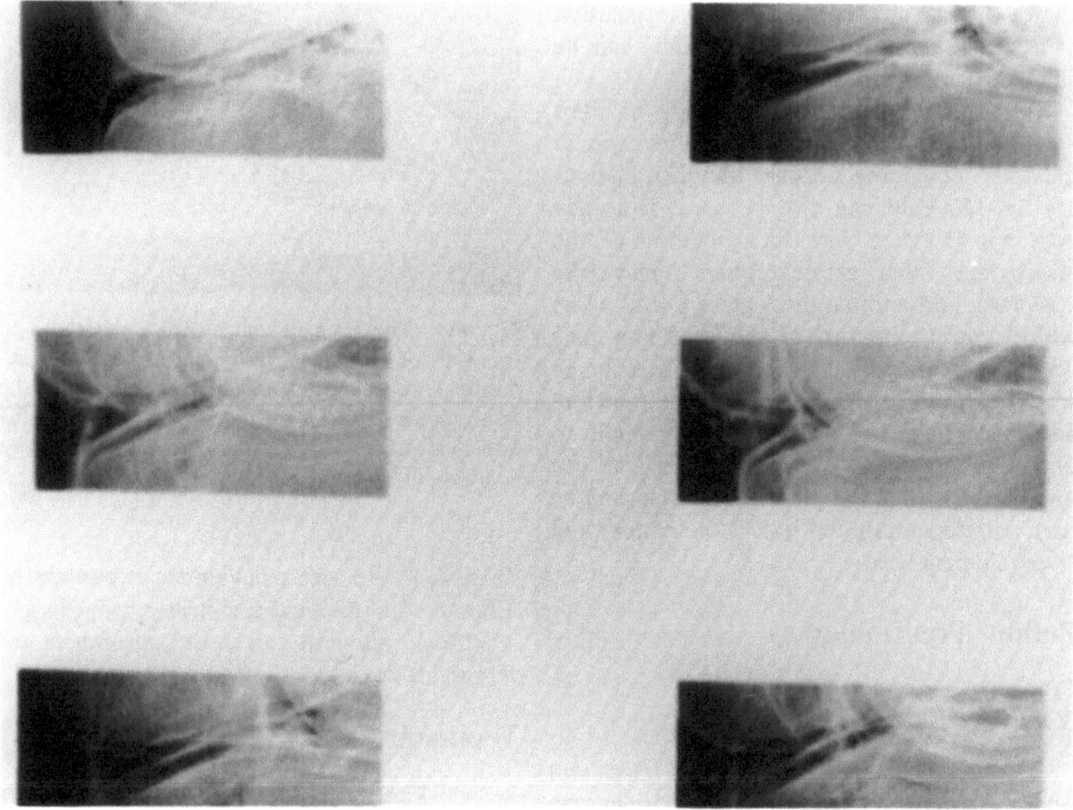

Fig. 41. Six exposures of the normal body and posterior horn of the lateral meniscus were obtained on one 9 × 9-in. film.

tella or femoral condyles, and this should be avoided if possible.

Intraarticular positioning of the needle is easy if there is synovial effusion because the suprapatellar pouch is distended. If there is no synovial effusion the suprapatellar pouch is collapsed, and positioning of the needle is slightly more difficult, but it usually does not present a major problem.

Aspiration of synovial fluid confirms the intraarticular position of the needle. Any fluid within the joint should be aspirated completely, if possible, to avoid dilution of the contrast material in the joint. If no fluid is aspirated, 5–10 cc air should be injected through the needle. The air should flow freely into the joint without resistance, and it should be possible to easily aspirate it back into the syringe. If the injected air cannot be aspirated easily it usually means that the needle is extraarticular. The needle should then be withdrawn partially

and reinserted until air can be injected and aspirated.

If there is any question about the intraarticular position of the needle a test injection of 0.5 contrast material should be made, and the flow of contrast material into the joint should be observed under fluoroscopy. If the needle is intraarticular, contrast material will flow away from the tip and will usually pool in the lateral recesses of the joint (Fig. 44). If the needle is extraarticular, contrast material will not flow away from the tip and will infiltrate the extraarticular soft tissues around it (Fig. 45). A total of 4–6 cc of 60% or 76% meglumine diatrizoate or iothalamate is used.

Immediately after injection of contrast material, 30–40 cc of room air is injected into the joint. The injection of air causes distension of the joint capsule and patients usually complain of a tight feeling in the knee. The patient should then sit on the table with the legs

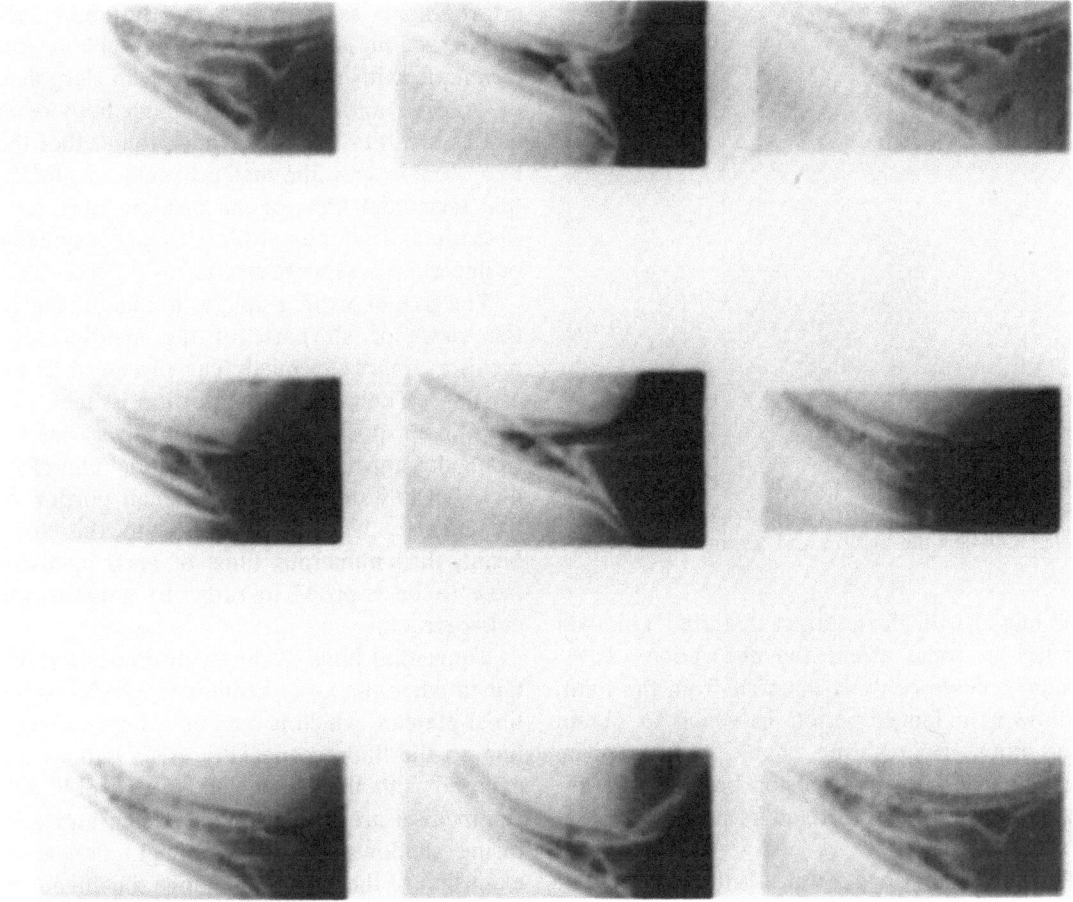

Fig. 42. Nine exposures of a torn medial meniscus were obtained on the 9 × 9-in. spot film.

dangling over the edge. The knee should be flexed and extended passively for about 20–30 s in order to spread the contrast material around the joint.

Extraarticular injections of contrast material should be rare if proper positioning of the needle is tested by injection and aspiration of air, and if fluoroscopy is used to observe the flow of contrast medium if any uncertainty exists. Intraarticular injection of water-soluble contrast material is painless. Any complaint of pain during the injection of contrast material should raise the suspicion of extraarticular injection. If contrast material has been injected extraarticularly the knee should be observed fluoroscopy. If the contrast material overlies the joint space it will obscure the menisci, and the procedure should be rescheduled for another day. However, it usually will be well above the joint space and will not interfere with eval-

uation of the menisci. Contrast material and air may be immediately reinjected and the arthrogram obtained.

Water-soluble contrast material is rapidly absorbed from the knee, but 2–3 days is required for air to be absorbed. Therefore the patient should be warned that mild discomfort may be experienced in the knee for 2–3 days after arthrography. No specific limitation of activities is necessary because of the procedure. The splashing sound heard in the knee is due to air and fluid and is of no significance.

Carbon dioxide has been used instead of room air because it is absorbed rapidly and will shorten the period of discomfort. We found, however, that it was a burden to maintain the equipment for injection of carbon dioxide, and so we have used ordinary room air without any serious problem.

A dose of 0.3 cc epinepherine 1:1000 can

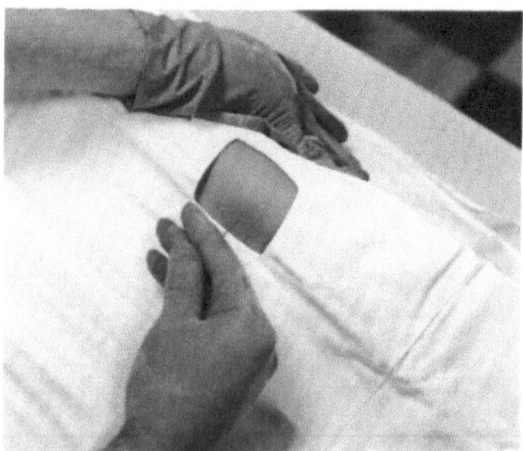

Fig. 43. The joint is punctured with a 20-gauge needle placed beneath the midportion of the patella between the patella and femoral condyles.

be mixed with the contrast material. This will delay to some extent the absorption of the water-soluble contrast material from the joint, allowing a longer period in which to obtain the films. Epinephrine should not be given to patients with hypertension because it is absorbed into the bloodstream from the synovium.

Fluoroscopic Spot Film Method. We use the fluoroscopic spot-film method of knee

arthrography as described by Butt and McIntyre, and no longer use the cross-table lateral technique with the horizontal beam described by Andren and Wehlin. Although both techniques are satisfactory we have found that the fluoroscopic spot-film method enables us to obtain tangential films of the menisci more consistently and additional films of any suspicious or uncertain area more easily.

The goal of arthrography is to obtain tangential views of all parts of the menisci. The menisci are two semicircular pieces of fibrocartilage. Their peripheral portion is thick and their inner portion thin, which gives them a triangular appearance on a tangential film (Fig. 46). On any one film only a small portion of the menisci will be tangential to the x-ray beam; thus numerous films of each meniscus have to be exposed in order to visualize the entire structure.

Tangential films of the menisci are best obtained when the x-ray beam is tangential to the tibial plateau, which is seen as a single straight line on the fluoroscope (Fig. 47). If films are exposed with the tibial plateau seen obliquely the menisci are not adequately seen, and confusing shadows may result. Slight flexion or extension of the knee will change the alignment of the tibial plateau, and the films should be

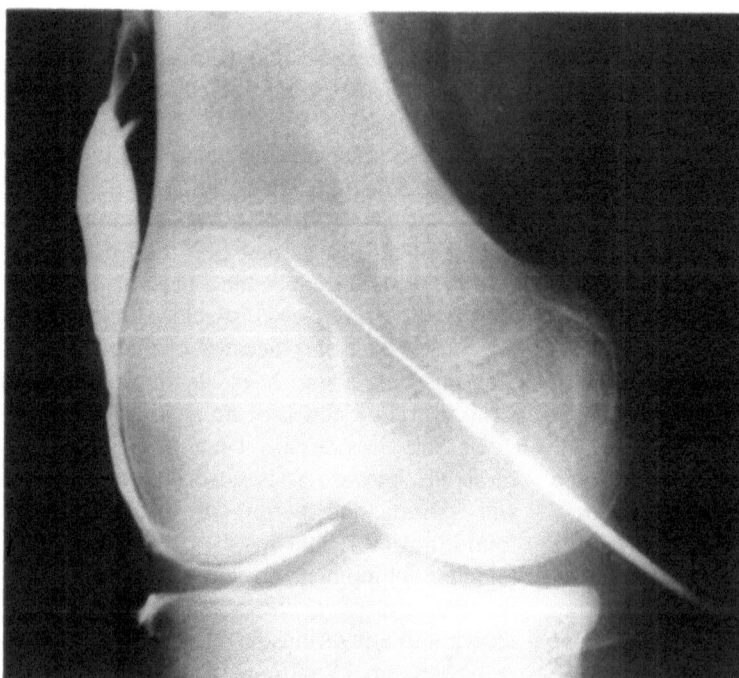

Fig. 44. With an intraarticular injection, fluoroscopy should show the contrast material flowing away from the tip of the needle and into the lateral aspect of the joint capsule.

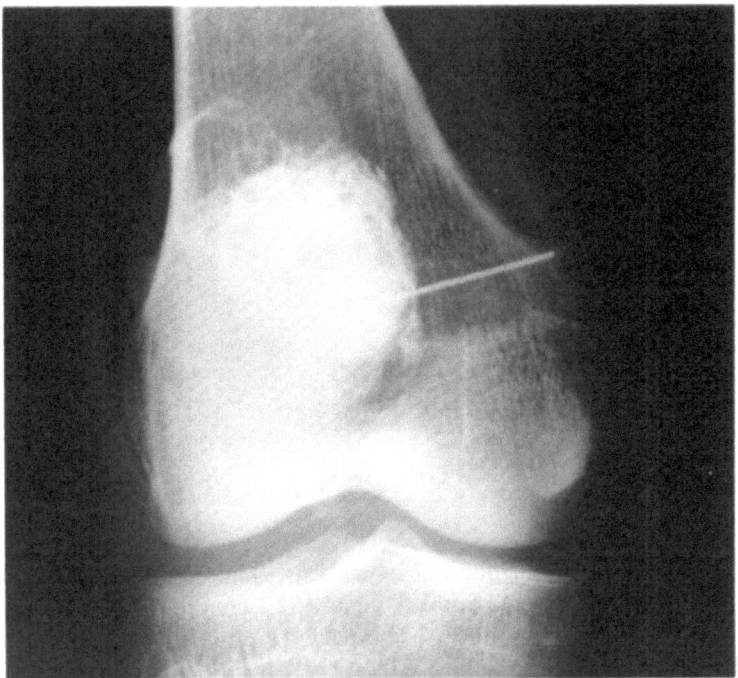

Fig. 45. If the needle is extraarticular, contrast material will stay around the tip and infiltrate the extraarticular soft tissues.

exposed only when the tibial plateau is seen in tangent.

In the method we describe here the left hand of the radiologist works the tower with the spot-film device, while the right hand is placed around the patient's ankle or foot in order to turn the leg and apply the stress to the knee. The image intensifier should be brought as close to the knee as possible so as to reduce magnification artifact. Motion artifact also degrades film image; it can be reduced by having as short an exposure time as possible and by keeping the patient's knee and the fluoroscopic tower steady while the film is being exposed.

Left Medial Meniscus (from the Anterior to Posterior Horn). The medial meniscus is usually photographed first since it is torn much more frequently than the lateral meniscus.

Patient Positioning

Prone
Tibia abducted
Later, 45° left anterior oblique with left side against fluoroscopic table

Film Sequence

Total: 12 films

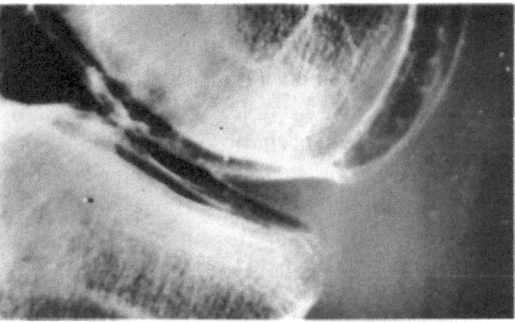

Fig. 46. The x-ray beam is tangential to the body of the medial meniscus. Because the peripheral portion of the meniscus is thick and there is a thin inner portion, the meniscus has a triangular configuration on a tangential view.

Technique

With the patient prone on the fluoroscopic table, the sling is placed around the thigh just above the knee, and the hook is slid beneath the opposite leg and attached to the side of the table opposite the leg that is being filmed. Abduction of the tibia will allow valgus stress to be applied with widening of the medial compartment of the knee joint. The stress separates the meniscus from the tibial plateau and femoral condyle and also enables the air and con-

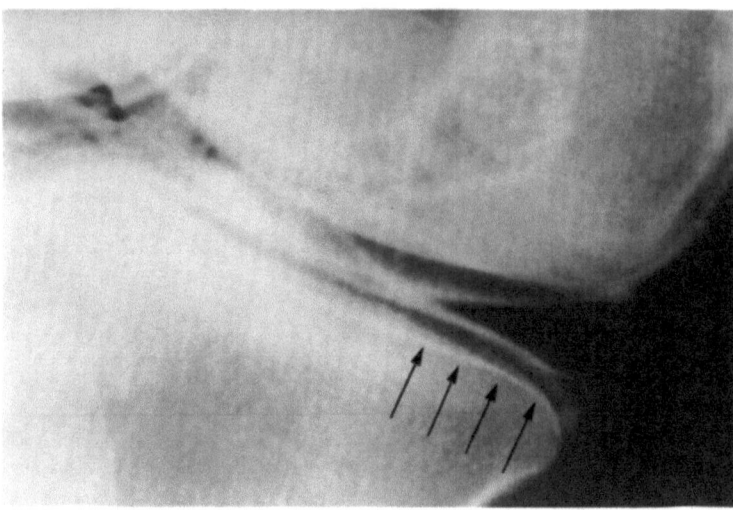

Fig. 47. The menisci are best seen when the x-ray beam is tangential to the tibial plateau. The anterior and posterior portions of the tibial plateau are superimposed and appear as a single straight line (*arrows*).

trast material to surround the meniscus. The patient is then rotated into about a 45°, left anterior oblique position with the patient's left side against the fluoroscopic table.

The examiner's hand grasps the patient's foot or ankle and turns it to the left (Fig. 48a). On fluoroscopy, the knee should be seen in a steep oblique position (Fig. 48b). The knee should not be in a completely lateral position as this will just superimpose the medial and lateral menisci on each other. Valgus stress should be applied and the knee should be manipulated with slight flexion and extension until the tibial plateau is seen in tangent and the first film should be exposed. The ankle or

foot is then rotated toward the right so that the femoral condyles move about 10–15° and the second exposure made. There is continued rotation of the patient toward the left with movement of the femoral condyles 10–15° so that by the time the sixth film is being exposed the patient is lying flat on his stomach and the knee is seen in a directly PA projection (Fig. 49).

Another film is inserted and six more exposures are obtained with continued rotation of the knee and patient's body towards the right. The last film should be obtained with the lateral femoral condyle just superimposed on the inner margin of the posterior horn of

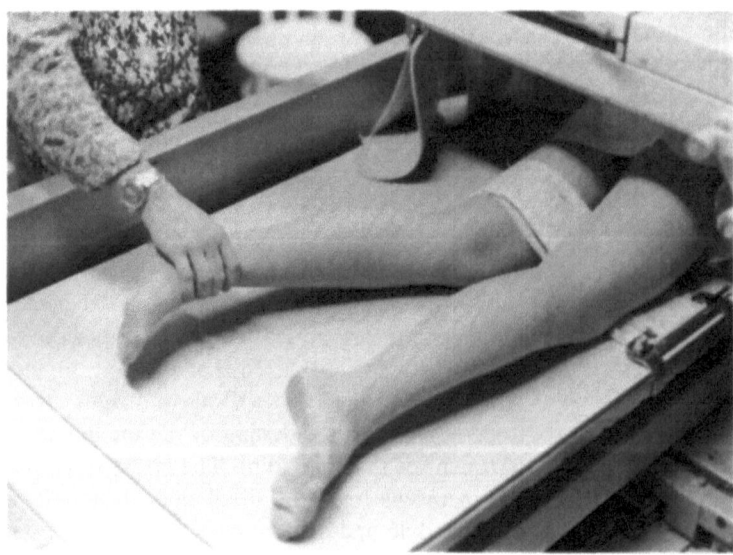

Fig. 48a. Photographing the anterior horn of the medial meniscus. The sling is placed just above the left knee and attached to the right side of the table. The patient is turned into a moderate left anterior oblique position, and the foot and ankle are turned to the left.

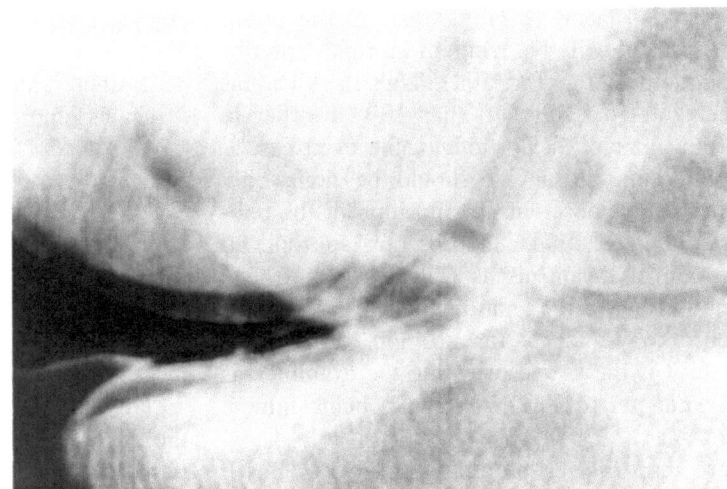

Fig. 48b. The anterior horn is seen with the knee in a steep left anterior oblique position. The femoral condyles are overlapping but are not completely superimposed.

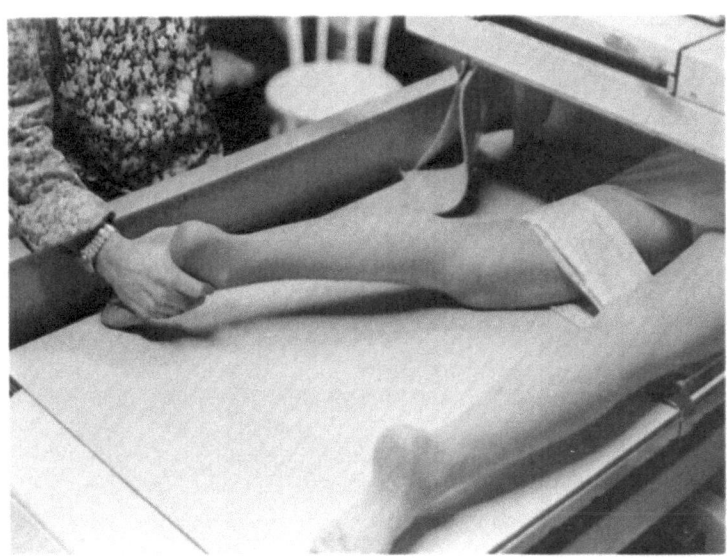

Fig. 49a. Filming the body of the medial meniscus. The patient is lying on her stomach. Valgus stress is being applied to widen the medial compartment of the knee joint.

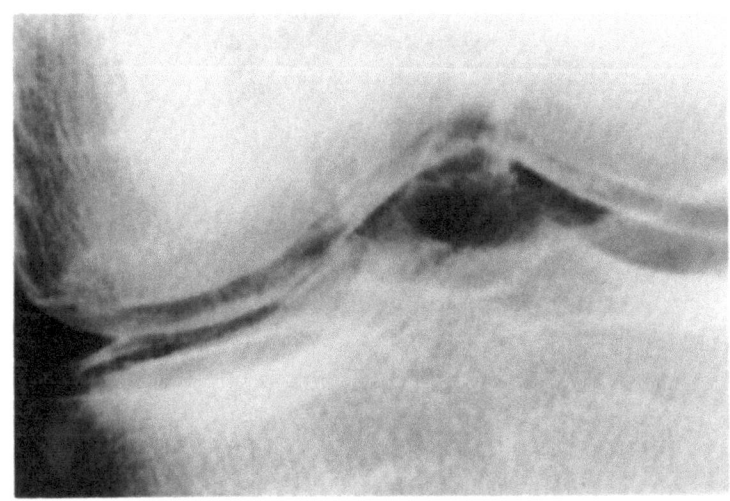

Fig. 49b. The body or midportion of the medial meniscus is seen when the knee is in a straight PA projection.

the medial meniscus (Fig. 50b). At this point, the patient will be lying in a right anterior oblique position (Fig. 50a). Thus the knee has been rotated a little less than 180° in order to obtain films of all portions of the meniscus.

Rotation of the leg should be done only when one is observing the position of the femoral condyles under fluoroscopy so that no portion of the meniscus will be skipped. The relationship of the femoral condyles as seen on fluoroscopy and not the position of the ankle or foot is the key in orienting the examiner as to what part of the meniscus is being filmed.

Left Lateral Meniscus (Anterior Horn). The lateral meniscus is filmed next.

Patient Positioning

45° right anterior oblique with right side against fluoroscopic table (Fig. 51)

Film Sequence

Total: 12 films

Technique

The sling is removed and replaced around the thigh again but with the hook reattached to the table on the same side as the knee that is being filmed, so that with adduction of the

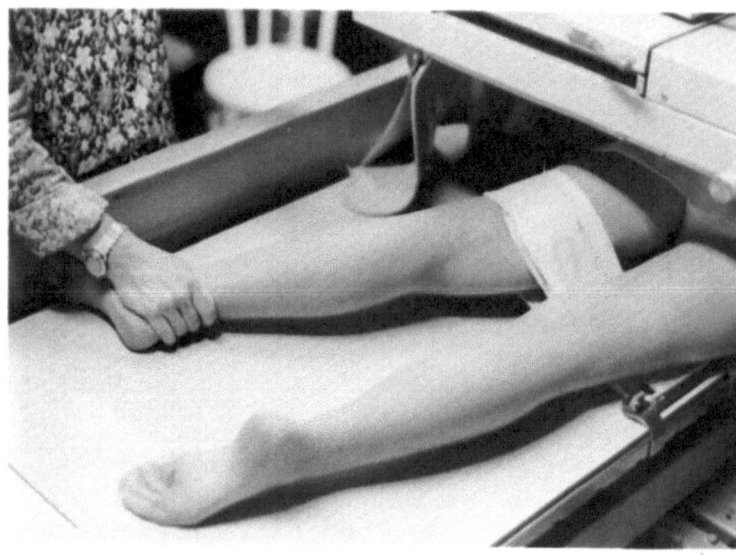

Fig. 50a. Filming the posterior horn of the left medial meniscus. The patient is turned into a moderate right anterior oblique position, and the foot and ankle are turned all the way to the right.

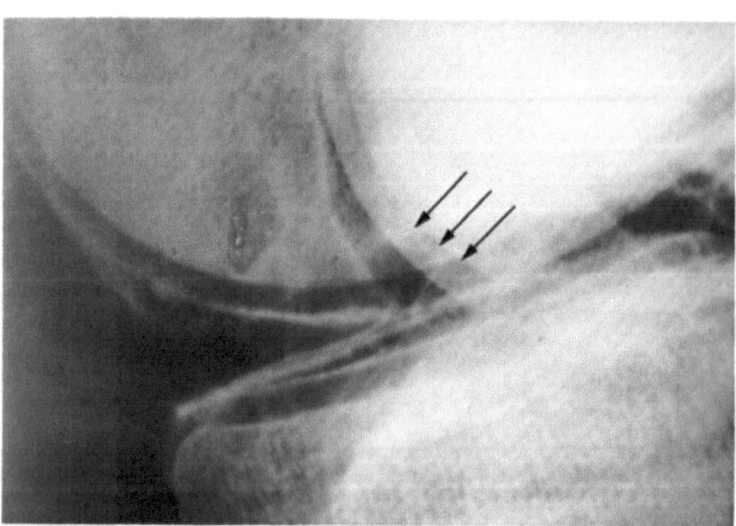

Fig. 50b. The posterior horn is seen with the knee in a steep right anterior oblique position. The lateral femoral condyle (*arrows*) almost overlaps the inner border of the posterior horn of the medial meniscus.

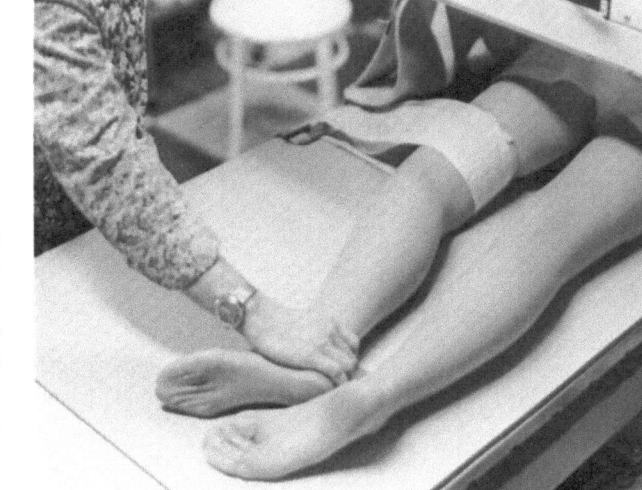

Fig. 51a. Filming the anterior horn of the left lateral meniscus. The patient is turned into the right anterior oblique position and the foot is turned to the right. The sling is placed above the knee and attached to the left side of the table so that varus stress can be applied to widen the lateral compartment of the knee joint.

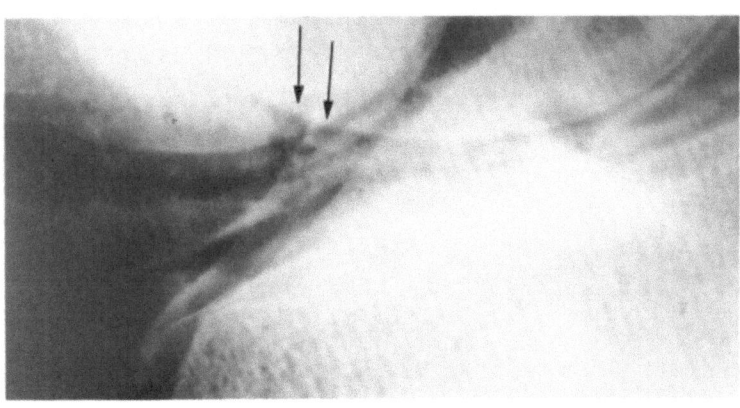

Fig. 51b. The anterior horn is seen with the knee in a steep right anterior oblique position. The medial femoral condyle (*arrows*) almost overlaps the inner border of the anterior horn of the lateral meniscus.

tibia varus stress will applied to the knee. In a similar manner as was done for the medial meniscus, the patient's knee is rotated 10–15° toward the left for each exposure and 12 spot films are obtained of the lateral meniscus Figs. 52 and 53).

The sling is then removed and the patient is placed in the left lateral position and the left knee is flexed 60–80°; exposure is made 8 kv higher than the initial exposure and a lateral spot film of the entire knee is obtained (Fig. 54). This allows visualization of the cruciate ligaments and the joint capsule. Another film is then inserted and views of the patellar cartilage are obtained (Fig. 55a). In the straight lateral position with the leg extended and with slight external rotation, the lateral facet of the patella cartilage will come into view (Fig. 55b). With slight internal rotation, the medial facet is observed (Fig. 55c).

If there is a suspicion of cruciate ligament tear, an additional cross-table lateral film is obtained with the overhead tube. The patient sits on the end of the fluoroscopic table with the knee flexed 90° and with the lower leg hanging over the edge of the table. A grid cassette is held by the patient between the knees and an overpenetrated cross-table lateral view of the knee is obtained (Fig. 56a). This allows the contrast material to pool over the synovial reflection of the cruciate ligaments (Fig. 56b).

After each film is exposed it should be immediately taken to the dark room and developed by a rapid film processor. The radiologist should have films available for review as soon as the procedure is finished. This will allow

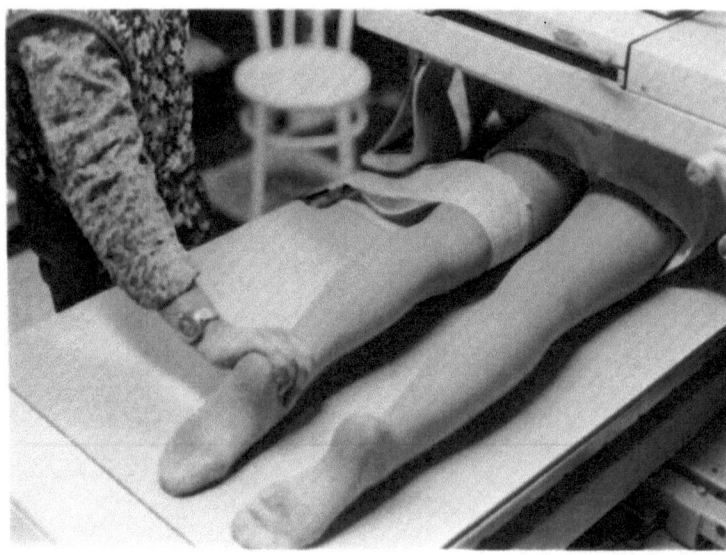

Fig. 52a. Filming the body of the lateral meniscus. The patient is flat on her stomach, and the knee and foot are in a straight PA projection.

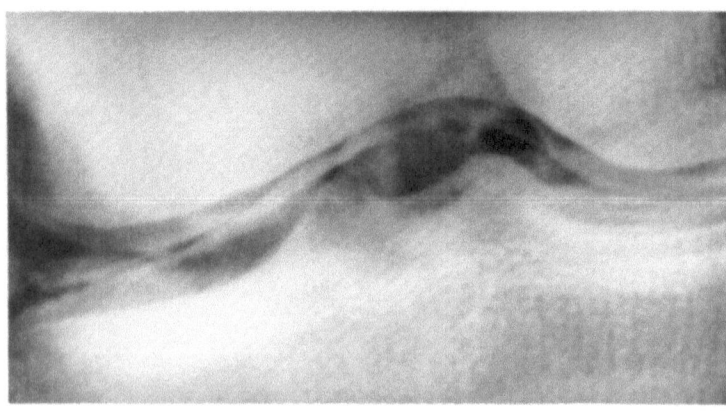

Fig. 52b. The body of the lateral meniscus is seen with the knee in a straight PA projection.

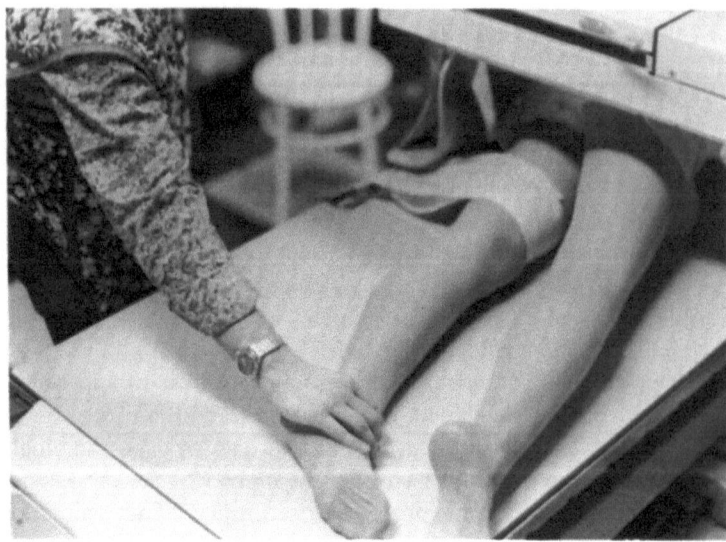

Fig. 53a. Filming the posterior horn of the left lateral meniscus. The patient is turned into the left anterior oblique position with the foot and ankle turned to the left.

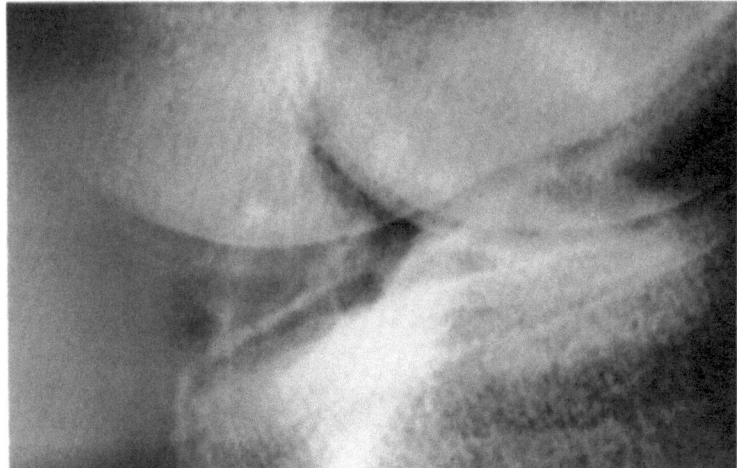

Fig. 53b. The posterior horn is seen with the knee in a steep left anterior oblique position with the medial femoral condyle almost overlapping the inner border of the meniscus.

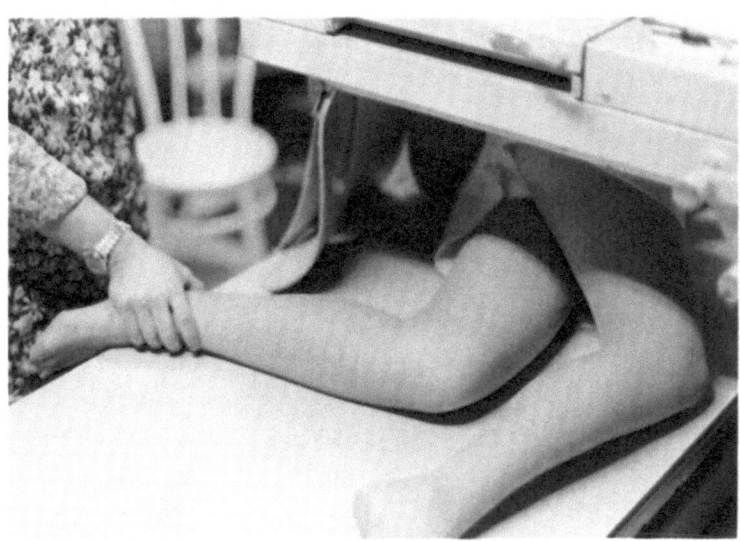

Fig. 54a. Obtaining a full lateral spot film of the knee. The knee is flexed 60°–90°.

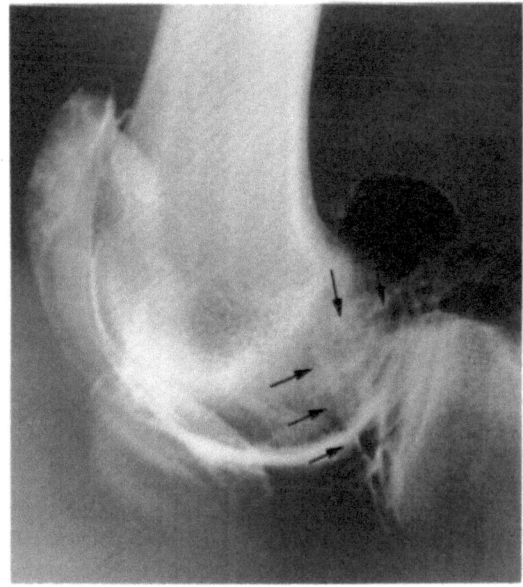

Fig. 54b. The lateral spot film shows the normal anterior and posterior cruciate ligaments (*arrows*) and the joint capsule.

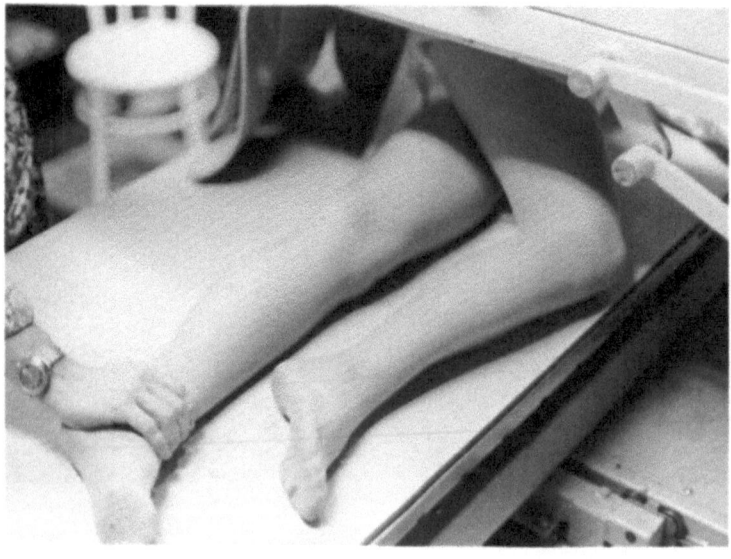

a

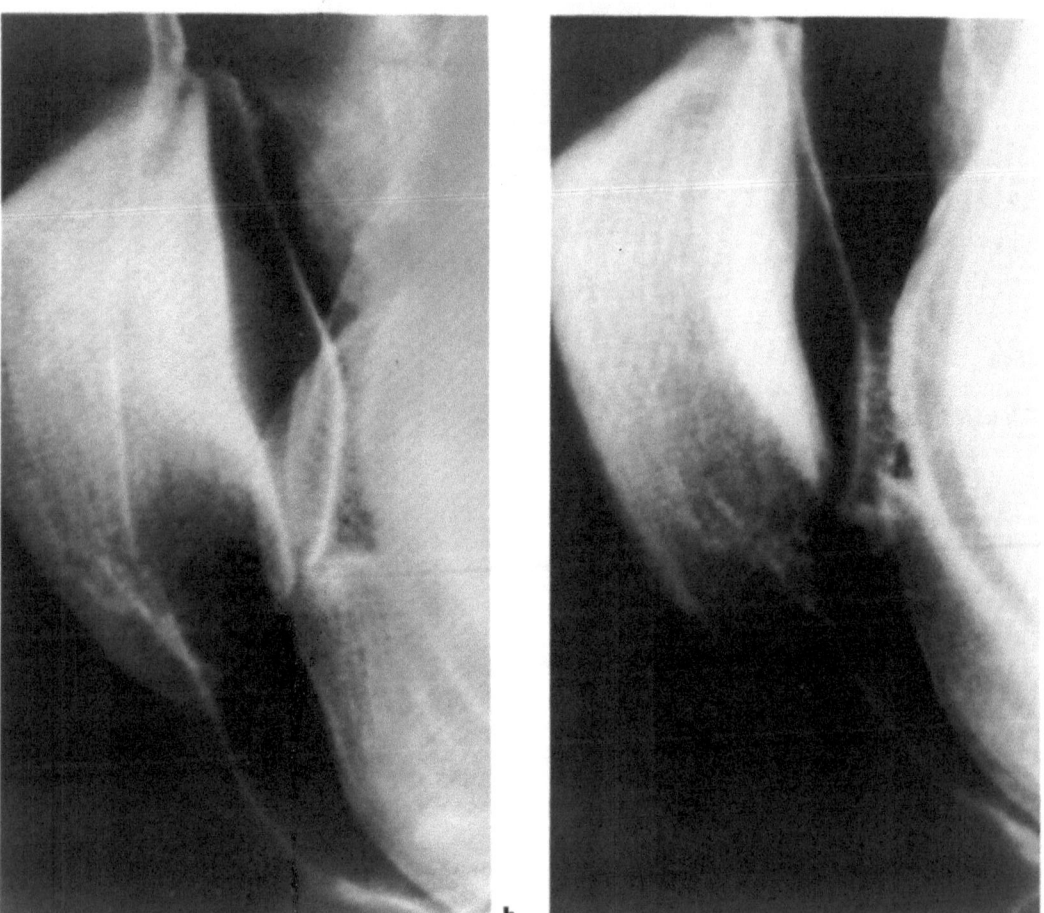

b   c

Fig. 55, a–c. Visualization of the patellar cartilage. **a** A lateral spot film is obtained with the knee extended. **b** With mild external rotation the lateral facet of the patellar cartilage is seen. **c** With slight internal rotation the medial facet of the patellar cartilage comes into view.

any suspicious or inadequately seen areas to be photographed. The contrast material is rapidly absorbed from the knee joint, and after about 30 min, adequate detail of the menisci can no longer be obtained. The entire procedure, including injection and filming, should take approximately 20–30 min.

Shoulder Arthrography

Pain and limitation of motion of the shoulder may be caused by many different soft-tissue abnormalities. The diagnosis cannot always be made with assurance by history, physical examination, and plain radiographs. Shoulder

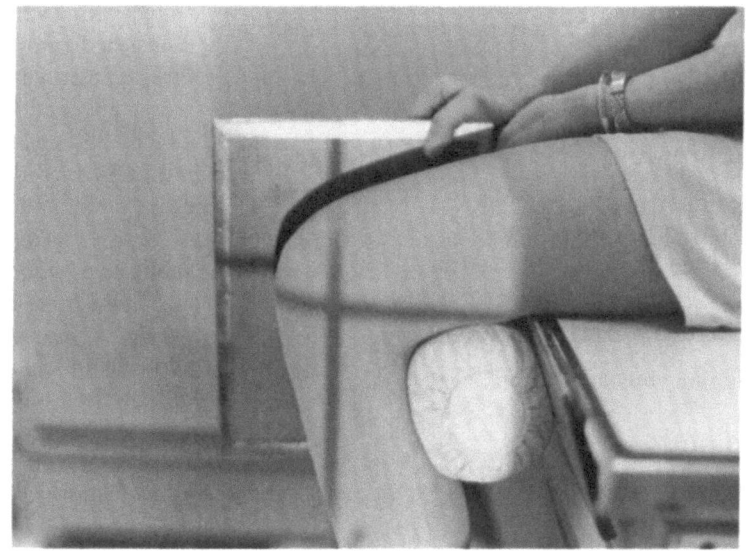

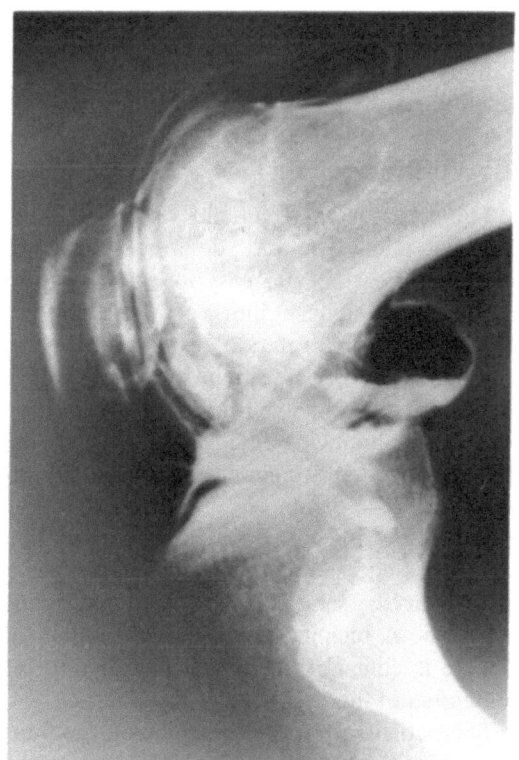

Fig. 56, a and **b.**   Visualization of the cruciate ligaments. **a** A Cross-table lateral view with the knee flexed 90° and with a cushion behind it is obtained with the overhead tube. **b** On the cross-table lateral view the ligaments are seen as the contrast material layers over their synovial reflection.

arthrography is rarely requested in patients with calcific peritendinitis because tears of the rotator cuff are uncommon in this situation.

Purpose

To aid in diagnosis of:
 Tear of rotator cuff
 Frozen shoulder
 Capsular deformity due to previous dislocation
 Dislocation of biceps tendon

Equipment

Standard arthrography tray
20- or 22-gauge 3.5-in. disposable spinal needle
Lead O marker

Patient Positioning

Supine with shoulder flat against table

Injection

Total of 10–12 cc

Position

Internal rotation view
External rotation view
Axillary view
Bicipital-groove view

Technique

There are several techniques for injecting the shoulder joint. The one described here has been found to be safe, easy to learn, easy to perform. Preliminary films of the shoulder, including internal rotation, external rotation, and axillary views, are obtained and reviewed. For the internal and external rotation views the x-ray tube should be tilted about 20° in the caudad direction to increase the space seen between the acromion and humeral head. The axillary view is most easily obtained with a curved cassette; however, if none is available, an ordinary cassette can provide a good axillary view. A bicipital-groove view is obtained if there is clinical suspicion of abnormality of the tendon of the long head of the biceps.

The patient is positioned supine on the fluoroscopic table. With the aid of fluoroscopy, the marker is placed over the glenohumeral joint at the junction of the middle and lower thirds (Fig. 57). This point is marked on the skin with an indelible felt-tip marker. The patient should be cautioned not to move the arm or shoulder even slightly, or the mark may no longer correspond to the glenohumeral joint. The shoulder is scrubbed with povidone-iodine and draped. The skin beneath the mark is infiltrated with 1–2 cc lidocaine. The spinal needle is inserted into the skin beneath the mark and directed straight down toward the glenohumeral space (Fig. 58). As the needle is advanced its position should be checked intermittently with the fluoroscope. If the needle is not exactly overlying the glenohumeral space or if it is deviated into an oblique position, it should be withdrawn partially or completely and reinserted until it is vertical and exactly overlying the glenohumeral space. If needed, additional local anesthetic can be given through the needle.

The glenohumeral joint is relatively deep, and if the needle meets resistance after passing only a short distance through the skin, it is probably striking the humeral head. With a directly vertical approach the correct medial-to-lateral position of the needle is determined by fluoroscopy. The depth of the joint is still not known; however, this does not present any problem. If the needle is overlying the glenohumeral space when it meets resistance, it should be impinging on the articular cartilage of the glenoid. After meeting resistance the needle should be withdrawn 1–2 mm to free the tip from the underlying cartilage. Aspiration of the joint should be attempted, but fluid is not usually obtained from the shoulder. Lidocaine 1–2 cc should be injected through the needle with a 2-cc syringe. The lidocaine should flow freely and easily into the joint. If it does not, either the needle is embedded within the cartilage and should be withdrawn 1–2 mm more, or it is extraarticular and should be withdrawn and reinserted until the proper position is achieved.

To confirm the position of the needle, a test dose of 0.5 cc or less of meglumine diatrizoate or iothalamate should be injected. If the needle is intraarticular, contrast material will flow away from its tip into the joint cavity (Fig. 59). If the needle is extraarticular, contrast material will not flow away from the tip and will infiltrate the extraarticular soft tissues around the needle (Fig. 60). Small extraarticular test injections around the middle and lower portion of the glenohumeral joint will not interfere with subsequent interpretation of the arthrogram, but too many may obscure the glenohumeral space and make correct needle positioning difficult. When proper needle positioning has been confirmed, a total of 10–12 cc contrast material is injected into the joint. An average joint can easily accept 12 cc; in frozen shoulder, however, the joint capsule is contracted, and considerable pain may be experience after injection of 5–8 cc. When the patient complains of pain, no more contrast material should be injected.

After the injection the needle should be immediately removed and the shoulder rotated from the external to internal position once or twice to spread the contrast material around the joint capsule. Not too much motion of the shoulder should be allowed before the initial set of radiographs is obtained; extensive motion of the shoulder can distend the joint capsule, causing rupture of its weak points and making interpretation of the arthrogram difficult. Internal, and external rotation (Fig. 61a and b) and axillary views (Fig. 62) should be obtained without delay because contrast material is absorbed fairly rapidly. While the films are being developed in the rapid film processor, the patient's shoulder should be put through a full range of motion either actively or passively. The films should be reviewed as soon as they are developed, and if no abnormality is seen or if the diagnosis is uncertain, a postexercise set of films should be obtained.

There may be a moderate increase in pain in the shoulder after arthrography. It should be explained to the patient that pain due to the procedure itself usually disappears within 24 hours and that there are no lasting effects from the study.

Ankle Arthrography

Sprained ankle is a term that is used to include a wide range of soft-tissue injuries of the ankle from mild soft-tissue swelling to partial or complete tears of the ligaments. Clinical tests do not always distinguish ligamentous

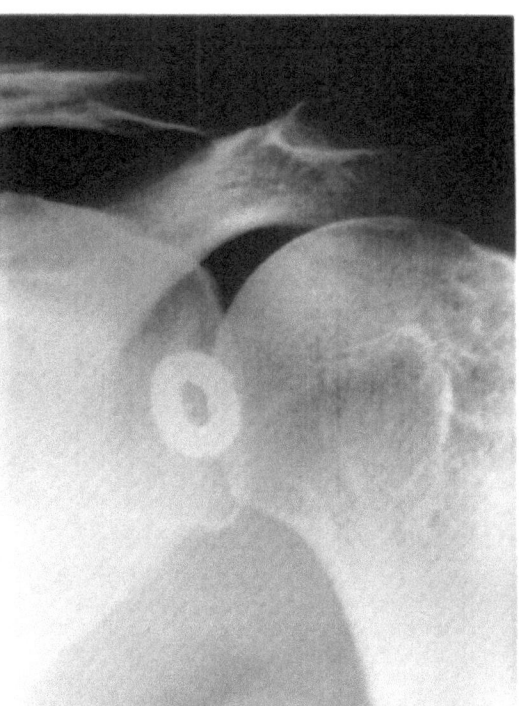

Fig. 57. Shoulder rotated into neutral to mild external rotation. A lead O marker is placed over the junction of the middle and lower thirds of the glenohumeral joint.

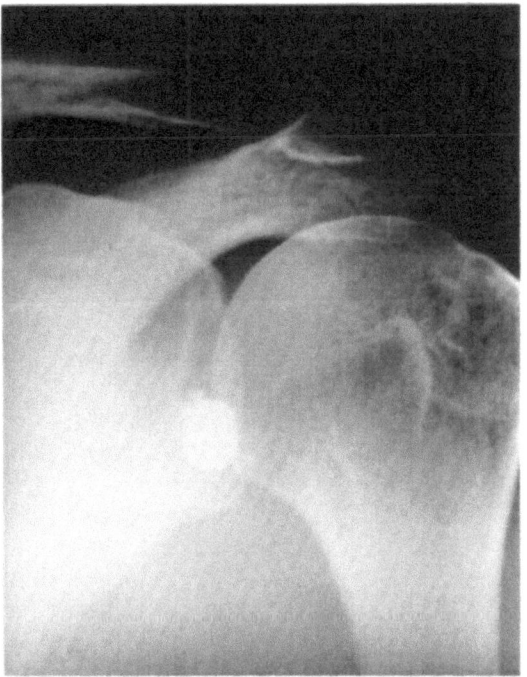

Fig. 58. Needle inserted into the skin and directed straight down toward the glenohumeral space.

tears from less serious soft-tissue injuries. Plain radiographs with stress views may not always demonstrate widening of the tibiotalar joint space after a ligament has ruptured, especially if there is severe pain and muscle spasm after the injury. With ankle arthrography, extravasation of contrast material out of the joint demonstrates ligamentous tear. Ankle arthrography should be done as soon as possible after injury because within 2–7 days the joint may become watertight, and the tear may not be demonstrated.

The number of requests for ankle arthrograms will depend to a large extent on the various methods of therapy used by the referring surgeons in their treatment of ankle sprains and osteochondritis dissecans.

Purpose

To demonstrate extent of soft-tissue injury

In osteochondritis dissecans:
    To determine if a loose fragment is present
    To determine if articular cartilage is intact
      or broken

Equipment

Standard arthrography tray
22-gauge 1.5-in. disposable needle
Lead O marker

Patient Positioning

Supine

Technique

After the patient is positioned on the fluoroscopic table the dorsalis pedis pulse is palpated and its position marked on the skin with an indelible felt-tip marker. The marker is placed a few millimeters below the tibiotalar joint, either slightly medial or lateral to the dorsalis pedis pulse (Fig. 63). This point is also marked on the skin with the indelible marker. The skin is scrubbed with povidone-iodine and draped. The skin beneath the mark is infiltrated with lidocaine. For the joint puncture the needle is inserted at the mark and directed slightly cephalad toward the tibiotalar joint. This cephalocaudal approach will allow the needle to avoid the anterior beak of the talus, which can prevent the needle from entering the joint if a directly vertical approach over the tibiotalar is used. After the needle has been inserted into the skin, the patient's ankle should be turned

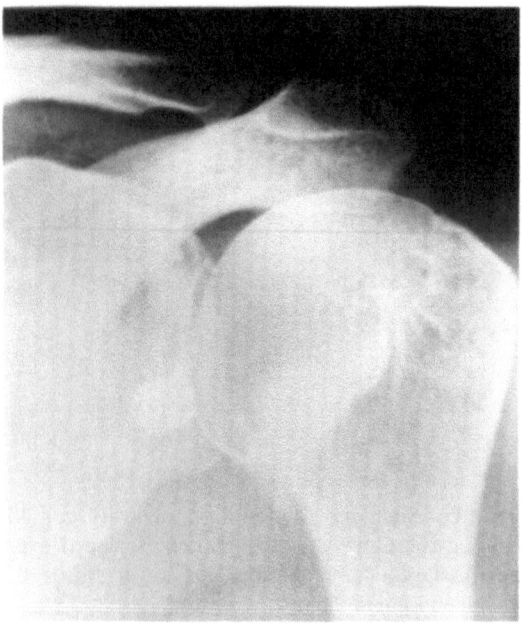

Fig. 59. Test injection showing contrast material flowing away from the tip of the needle and outlining the glenohumeral space and joint capsule.

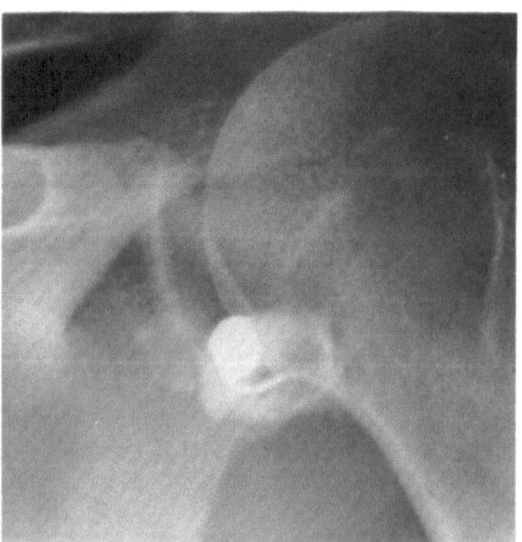

Fig. 60. Extraarticular test injection showing contrast material remaining around the tip of the needle rather than within the joint capsule.

into the lateral position and the location of the needle should be determined by fluoroscopy. With lateral fluoroscopy, the depth of the needle and its exact location with respect to the tibiotalar joint are easily seen. The needle should be advanced until it can be seen within the tibiotalar joint space (Fig. 64). If it is, 1 cc lidocaine injected through the needle should flow easily into the joint.

Single-contrast arthrography is used to demonstrate rupture of the ankle ligaments. A total of 5 cc meglumine diatrizoate or iothalamate is injected into the joint. With fluoroscopy, the contrast material should be seen to flow into the tibiotalar joint space. Contrast material may pool in the prominent anterior recess of the joint capsule. This should not be mistaken for extraarticular injection. The contrast material can extravasate out of the needle tract anteriorly if the joint is overdistended. After the needle is removed, AP, lateral and both oblique views of the ankle are obtained (Figs. 65 and 66). If no abnormality is seen or if diagnosis is uncertain, the ankle joint is put through a full range of motion and a post-exercise set of the same views is obtained.

Double-contrast arthrography is preferable to evaluate osteochondritis dissecans; 0.5 cc contrast material and 5–10 cc air should be injected. Tomograms may be used to supplement the plain films in determining whether the contrast material and air surround a loose osteocartilaginous fragment, which would in-

dicate that the articular cartilage is broken. Double-contrast arthrography is also helpful in differentiating between intraarticular loose bodies and extraarticular accessory ossicles around the ankle.

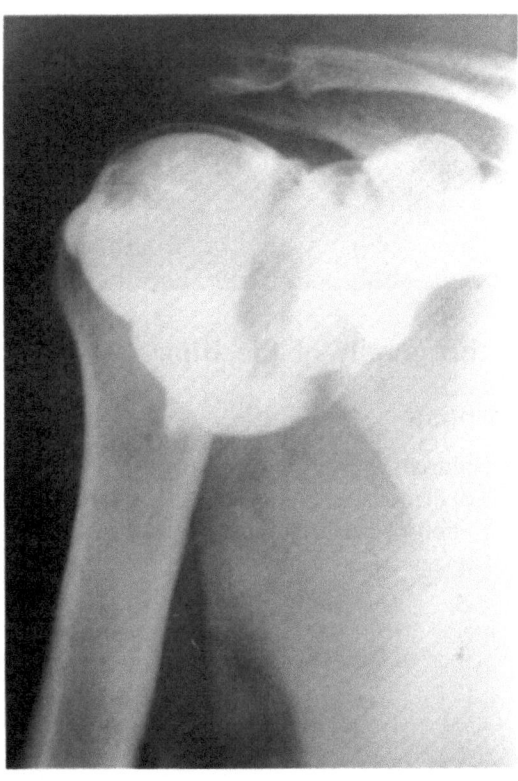

a

b

Fig. 61, a and **b**. Normal shoulder arthrogram. **a** Internal rotation view. **b** External rotation view.

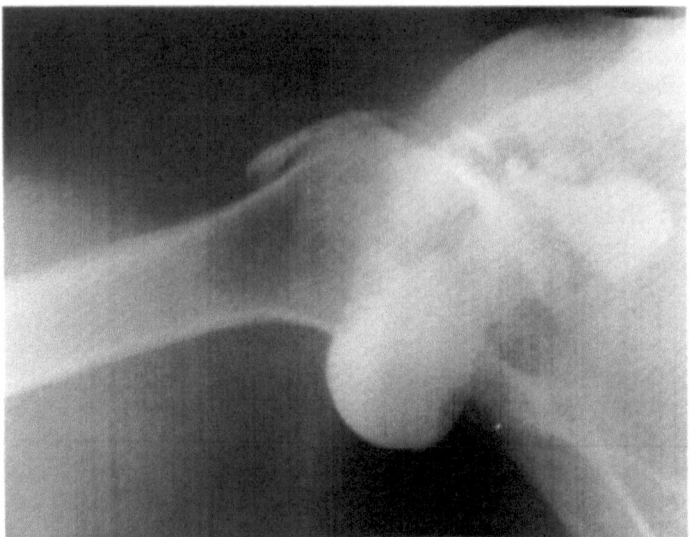

Fig. 62. Axillary view of normal shoulder arthrogram.

Arthrography of the Hip

Purpose

In children:

To demonstrate the size, shape, and position of cartilaginous femoral head

Congenital dislocation of hip: to determine

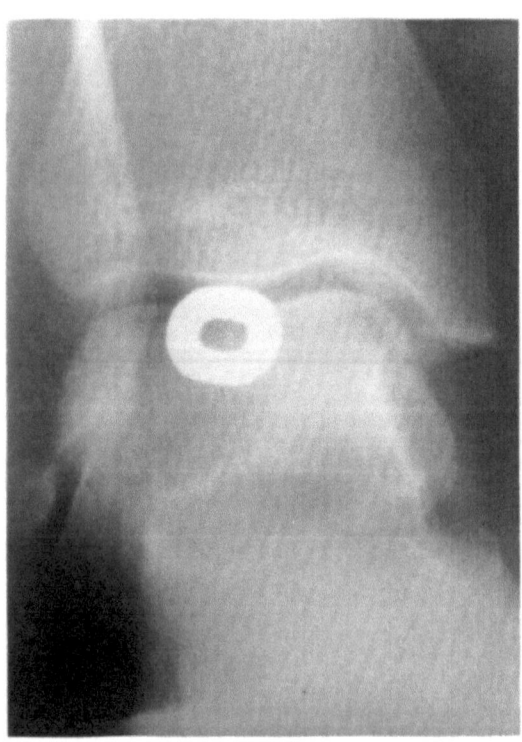

Fig. 63. Lead O marker slightly below the tibio-talar joint.

if limbus is inverted and position of femoral head

Legg-Perthes disease: to demonstrate shape of cartilaginous femoral head

Suspected septic arthritis of hip: to confirm position of needle in joint aspiration

In adults:

To evaluate total hip prosthesis

To demonstrate loose bodies in hip

To confirm position of needle in joint aspiration

Equipment

Standard arthrography tray

22-gauge 1.5-in. disposable needle (child)

20- or 22-gauge 3.5-in. disposable spinal needle (adult)

Patient Positioning

Supine

Technique

Injection of the hip in a child is somewhat more difficult than in an adult. Premedication is often needed so that the child will be sleeping when the procedure is performed. Careful observation is necessary after the procedure until sedation wears off. An infant is not difficult to control with one or two aides, and thus premedication is not needed. After the patient is positioned on the fluoroscopic table the

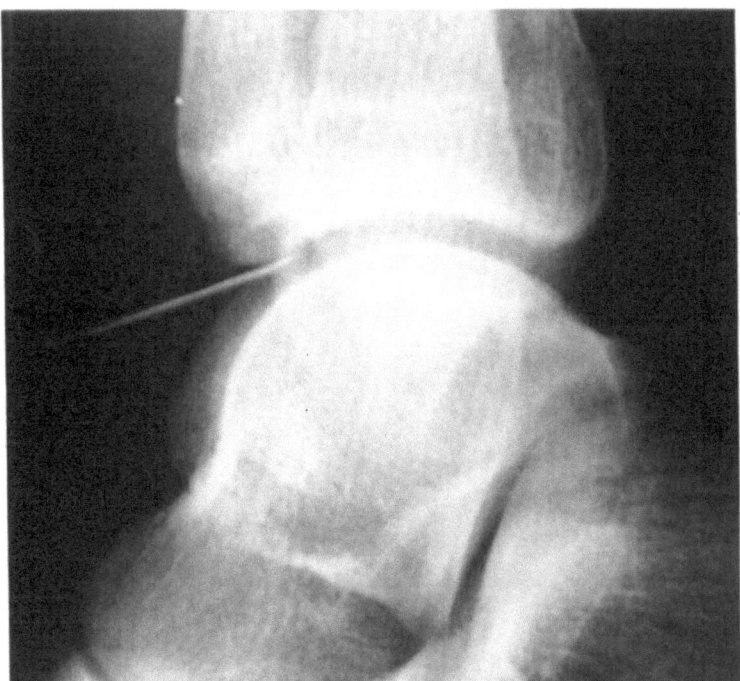

Fig. 64. Ankle turn into lateral position. Location of the needle in the tibiotalar joint is determined by fluoroscopy.

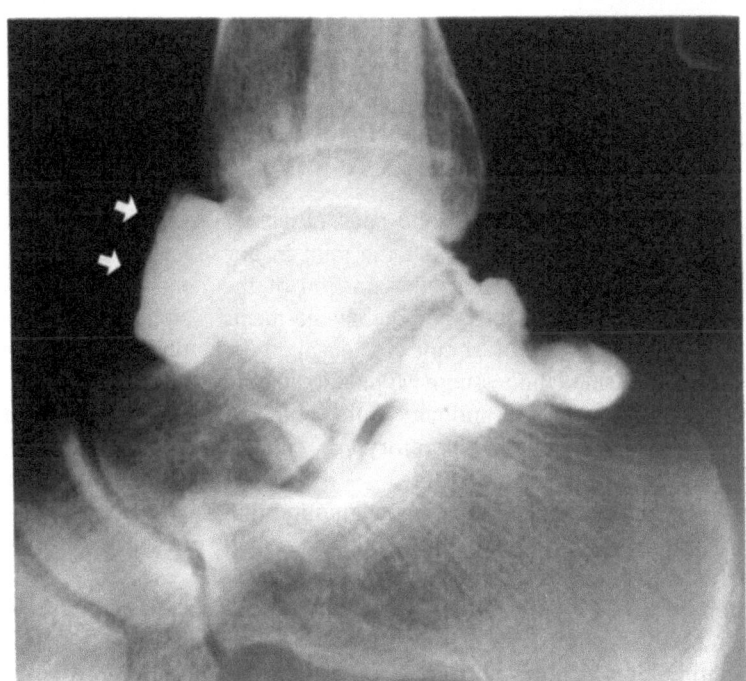

Fig. 65. Lateral view of normal ankle. Contrast material in the ankle joint and filling of the anterior recess of the joint (*arrows*) can be seen.

femoral artery is palpated and marked on the skin with an indelible felt-tip marker. The position of the femoral neck is ascertained by image-intensified fluoroscopy and marked on the skin. The groin is scrubbed with povidone-iodine and draped. Ordinarily local anesthesia is not necessary in infants or children, but is used in adults.

For the joint puncture in children the needle is inserted into the skin at a point slightly below the femoral neck and directed downward and cephalad toward the junction of the medial

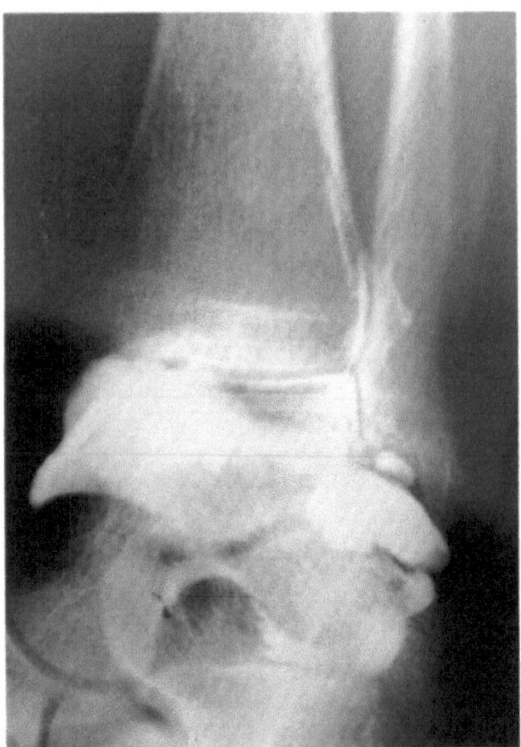

Fig. 66. Internal rotation view of normal ankle. Contrast material has not extravasated into the soft tissues around the ankle.

aspect of the femoral head and neck (Figs. 67 and 68). The needle can enter the joint in any position along the intracapsular portion of the femoral head and neck. When the needle meets resistance its position should be checked by image-intensified fluoroscopy. The hip should always be aspirated, and any fluid obtained should be sent to the laboratory for culture, sensitivity testing, and a smear.

The contrast material, 60% meglumine diatrizoate or iothalamate, is diluted to half strength with sterile saline or water for injection of the hip in children and is used full strength in adults. A few tenths of a cubic centimeter of contrast material should be injected to determine the position of the needle. If it is intraarticular the contrast material should flow away from the tip and outline the femoral head and hip joint (Fig. 69). In an infant only about 2 cc contrast material should be injected as too much will overdistend the joint, leading to leakage out of the needle tract. In an older child the amount is increased, and

in an adult a total of 10–12 cc is injected. After the needle is removed, AP and frog lateral radiographs of the hips should be obtained. The hip should then be put through a range of motion—internal and external rotation and abduction and adduction—to spread the contrast material around the joint, and after which another set of the same views should be obtained.

At the end of the procedure the groin should be checked for hematomas and the femoral pulse palpated; however, there have been very few complications from arthrography of the hip. There may be pain in the hip and radiating down the leg for several hours after the procedure as a result of distension of the hip joint capsule.

Arthrography of Hip Prostheses. Replacement of an arthritic hip joint with a total hip prosthesis is now a common surgical procedure. Despite the great success that has been achieved, in a small percentage of patients the prosthesis loosens or infection develops.

The commonly used total hip prostheses have acetabular and femoral components that are surrounded by methylmethacrylate cement. Barium is mixed with the cement so that it will become radiopaque. There normally is a thin area of lucency between the radiopaque cement and the bone. On an arthrogram, if contrast material is seen to enter the area of lucency it suggests that there is loosening of the prosthesis or abnormal binding at the cement-bone interface. Often, in a patient with hip pain, the joint is aspirated to obtain material for culture and sensitivity testing to rule out infection. At the same time as the aspiration, contrast material can be injected to determine if the prosthesis has loosened.

Equipment

Standard arthrography tray
20-gauge 3.5-in. disposable spinal needle

Patient Positioning

Supine

Technique

After the patient is positioned on the fluoroscopic table the femoral artery is palpated and its position marked on the skin with an indelible felt-tip marker. The position of the neck of the prosthesis is determined by image-intensified fluoroscopy and marked on the skin. The injection site should be about 4–5 fingerbreadths lateral to the femoral neck. The anterolateral approach is used rather than the straight vertical approach because the metallic femoral component of the prosthesis will obscure the metallic needle if they are superimposed. With the anterolateral approach, the tip of the needle can be visualized by fluoroscopy.

The skin at the injection site is infiltrated with lidocaine. The 20-gauge needle is inserted into the skin and directed downward and medially until it strikes the neck of the femoral component of the prosthesis (see Fig. 71). Intermittent fluoroscopy is used to determine if the needle is directed properly. The depth of the femoral neck can be determined only by trial and error. The sensation of the needle striking the metallic femoral neck can be distinguished from that of the needle striking bone or the polyethylene acetabular component. Mild flexion of the knee relaxes the joint capsule around the hip prosthesis and allows easier penetration of the needle beneath the joint capsule.

The hip joint should be aspirated and any fluid obtained sent to the laboratory for culture, sensitivity tests, and a smear. If no fluid is obtained, sterile saline is injected through the needle into the hip. A bacteriostatic agent is not used. If the needle is intraarticular the saline should flow relatively easily, although there may be slight resistance if the joint capsule around the prosthesis is contracted. The saline should be aspirated and sent to the laboratory for culture and sensitivity testing.

When the needle is in place an AP radiograph of the hip and entire prosthesis is obtained (Fig. 70). Immediately 10 cc 60% meglumine diatrizoate or iothalamate is injected and a second film obtained (Fig. 71). The patient's leg and hip must remain in exactly the same position for these two films. The needle is removed, and a frog lateral radiograph of the hip is obtained. The hip is then put through a full range of motion to spread the contrast material around the joint and a

second postexercise set of the same views is obtained.

With the injection of 10–12 cc contrast material there is usually distension of the tight joint capsule, which often causes hip pain and sometimes pain extending down the leg. At most, this usually disappears entirely several hours after the procedure.

The subtraction technique is used because the radiopaque methylmethacrylate is difficult to differentiate from the radiopaque contrast material (Fig. 72). Without the subtraction technique it is often difficult to determine if there is contrast material between the cement and the bone. This is the same subtraction technique used in angiography (see section, "Photographic Subtraction" in chapter, "General Considerations"). Special subtraction film is exposed through the scout film obtained with the needle in place but before the injection of contrast material. This is the reverse of the

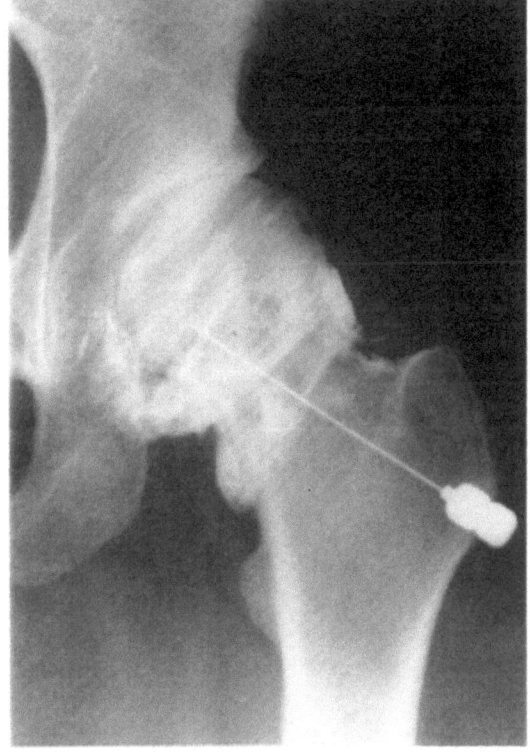

Fig. 67. A 20-gauge spinal needle inserted into the hip joint striking the bone at the junction of the femoral head and neck. Contrast material is seen within the hip joint capsule.

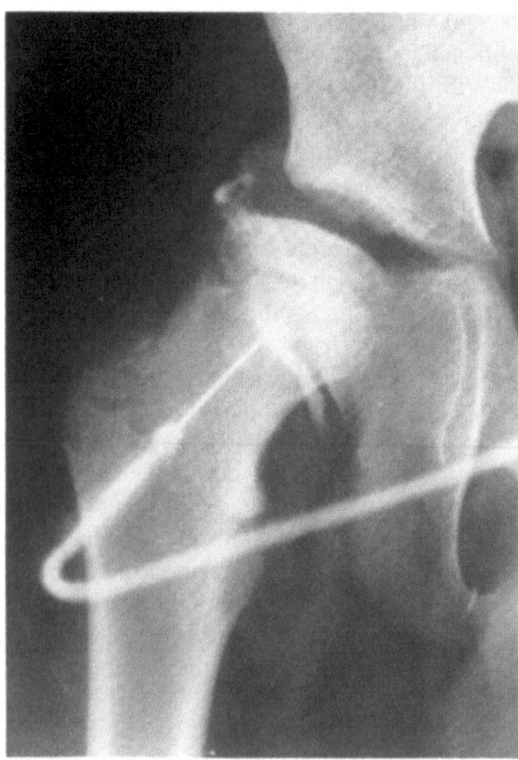

Fig. 68. Hip arthrogram of a 10-year-old boy with Legg-Perthes disease. The flow of contrast material into the hip joint can be observed on fluoroscopy if it is injected through sterile plastic tubing attaching the needle to the syringe.

scout film. This reversal film is then superimposed on the radiograph obtained just after the injection of contrast material. If there has been motion of the hip the two films may not superimpose exactly, which will lead to artifacts on the subtraction film. A duplication film is then made of the superimposed reversal film and the film with the contrast. On this duplication film the metal prosthesis, the methylmethacrylate, and the bone will be canceled out or subtracted and will appear gray; any contrast material will appear black. This readily shows if there is any contrast material between the cement and the bone (Fig. 72).

Wrist Arthrography

The wrist is divided into several noncommunicating compartments the major ones being the radiocarpal, radioulnar, and midcarpal joints. When arthrography shows abnormal communication between these joints it indicates that either arthritis or trauma has damaged the ligaments that separate them. Early in rheumatoid arthritis characteristic abnormalities seen on the arthrogram included a corrugated pattern of the synovium and communication between the various compartments

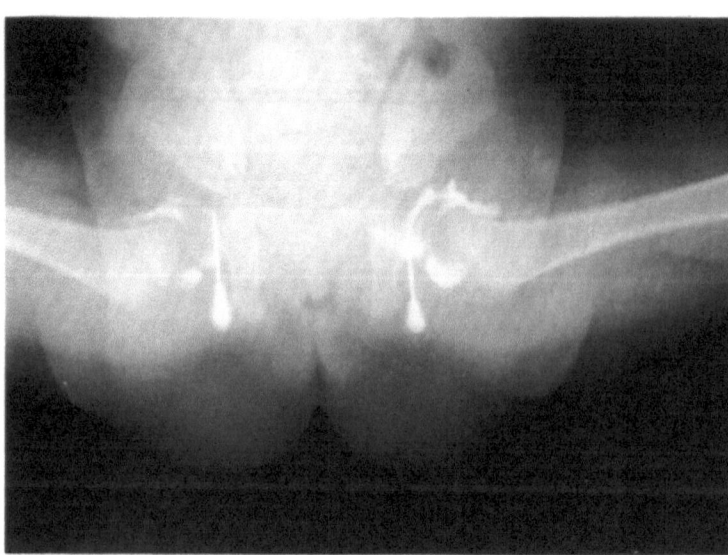

Fig. 69. Bilateral views of the hip in a child with bilateral congenital dislocation of the hips. The arthrogram shows that the dislocation has been reduced, the femoral heads being in normal position in relation to the acetabula.

of the wrist joint. These abnormalities were seen even in patients in whom the plain radiographs were normal. Despite this, wrist arthrography has rarely been requested to aid in the diagnosis of rheumatoid arthritis because this is usually based on clinical and laboratory findings. Its most frequent use has been in patients with wrist pain after trauma in whom plain films are normal.

Purpose

To study early changes of rheumatoid arthritis

To determine cause of wrist pain after trauma

To demonstrate tears of triangular cartilage separating radiocarpal from radioulnar joint

To demonstrate contrast material in ununited fracture of navicular bone

To diagnose synovial cysts communicating with joint

To show loose bodies within the joint

Equipment

Standard arthrography tray
Triangular foam-rubber sponge
25-gauge 0.75-in. needle
22-gauge 1.5-in. disposable needle

Technique

The patient sits in a chair beside a fluoroscopic table and places the affected hand and wrist palm down on the table. The wrist may be placed over a triangular foam-rubber sponge and flexed slightly to widen the radiocarpal joint. A lead marker is placed over the radiocarpal joint at the midportion of the navicular bone, and this point is marked on the skin with an indelible felt-tip marker. The puncture should not be made in the area between the navicular and lunate bones as the needle may inadvertently enter the midcarpal joint.

The injection site is scrubbed with povidone-iodine and draped. The skin is anesthetized with lidocaine. In some patients the joint may be entered with the 25-gauge needle while the skin is being anesthetized. In most patients, however, the joint must be punctured with the 22-gauge needle. The needle is inserted into the skin at the mark and directed downward toward the joint space (Fig. 73). If there is

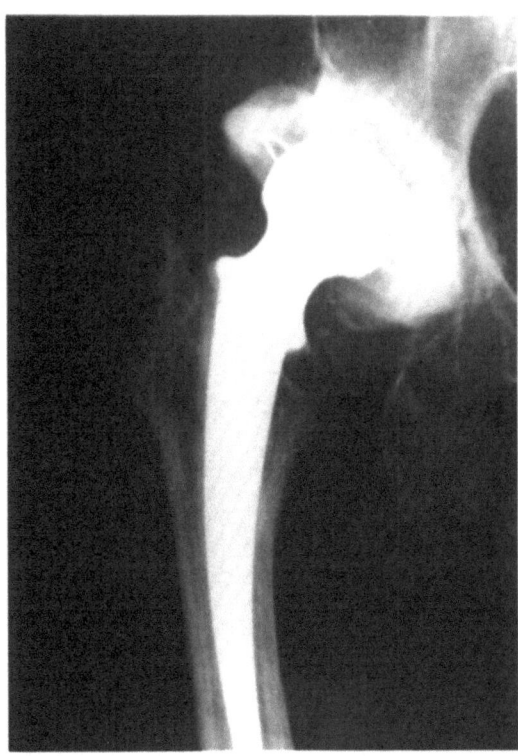

Fig. 70. Scout film showing the total prosthesis surrounded by radiopaque cement in good position in the right hip.

difficulty in placing the needle in the joint or uncertainty that it is in the proper position, the wrist should be turned into the lateral position to make fluoroscopic localization of the needle easier. Single-contrast arthrography is carried out with the injection of a total of 1.5–2 cc of 60% meglumine diatrizoate or iothalamate. If the wrist is normal fluoroscopy will show the contrast material flowing away from the needle tip and into the radiocarpal joint (Fig. 74). If the wrist is abnormal the contrast material may flow from the radiocarpal joint into the radioulnar or midcarpal joint (Fig. 75). After the needle is removed, AP, lateral, and oblique views of the wrist are obtained. No special precautions are necessary after wrist arthrography. Usually there is little or no additional discomfort because of the procedure.

Elbow Arthrography

Limitation of motion in the elbow may be due to loose bodies that arise from trauma or osteochondritis dissecans.

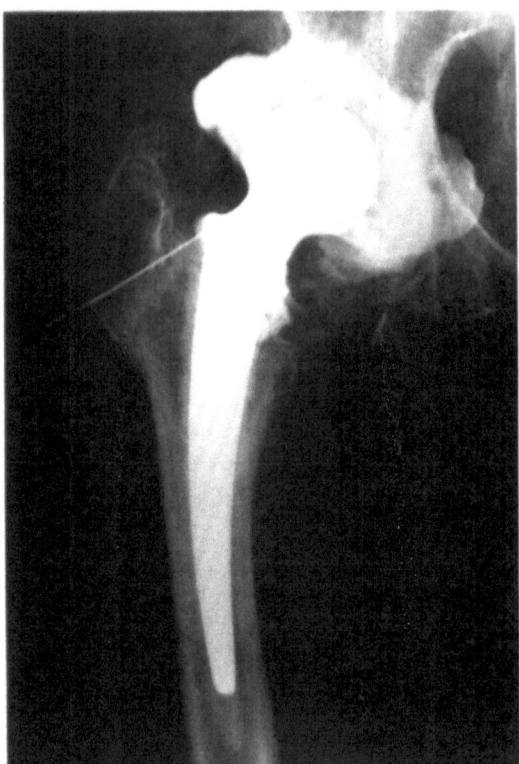

Fig. 71. Joint puncture with a spinal needle shown striking the metallic femoral neck. Contrast material was injected into the joint but is difficult to see because it is partially obscured by the radiopaque cement.

Purpose

To search for loose bodies within the joint

Equipment

Standard arthrography tray
22-gauge 1.5-in. disposable needle

Technique

The patient is placed on a chair or stool and rests the elbow in a lateral position on the fluoroscopic table. Three protuberances can be palpated with the elbow in this position: the olecranon process, lateral epicondyle, and radial head. These protuberances form the points of a triangle: the radial head and lateral epicondyle superior and the olecranon process inferior. Near the center of the triangle an opening can be palpated—the joint space between the radial head and capitullum. After the skin is anesthetized with a small amount of lidocaine, the needle is inserted laterally into the joint space just proximal to the radial head between the radial head and capitullum. The correct needle position above the radial head can be determined by fluoroscopy (Fig. 76).

Any fluid should be aspirated from the joint, following which 1 cc water-soluble contrast material and then 6–10 cc air are injected (Fig. 77), and the needle is removed. If too much air is injected the joint capsule will rupture, making the study difficult to interpret. AP, lateral, and oblique views and an upright lateral view of the elbow are obtained. The small amount of contrast material should give good coating of the articular cartilages around the elbow. Air should surround any radiolucent loose bodies, making them visible on the arthrogram (Fig. 78). Superimposition of the various structures of the elbow joint often makes interpretation of the arthrogram difficult. Tomography is often helpful in interpreting the arthrogram.

Lumbar Diskography

In diskography, contrast material is injected into the intervertebral disk itself. Often a patient with a degenerated or herniated disk is asymptomatic, and therefore diskography must always be correlated with the clinical symptoms before any treatment is given.

Purpose

To supplement myelography in evaluation of low-back pain that may be due to herniation of an intervertebral disk, e.g., when there is strong clinical evidence of disk herniation but the myelogram is normal or equivocal

To help localize the level of disk herniation when there is a discrepancy between the results of physical examination and the myelogram

To distinguish between extradural defects due to herniated disk and those due to other causes, including postsurgical scarring and metastatic tumor

Equipment

Myelography tray
Lead O markers
20-gauge 3.5-in. disposable spinal needles
25-gauge 5-in. spinal needles
Pillows or a large foam-rubber wedge

Patient Positioning

Prone

Technique

The transdural approach is the easiest to learn and perform, especially when biplane fluoroscopy is available. Posterolateral and lateral extradural approaches have also been developed, but only the transdural approach will be described here.

After the patient is positioned on the fluoroscopic table, pillows or the foam-rubber wedge should be placed beneath the abdomen to straighten or reverse the lordotic curve of the lumbar spine. This increases the space between the spinous processes and allows a greater degree of manipulation of the needles. Biplane fluoroscopy, although not absolutely necessary, makes performance of diskography much easier. A portable C-arm fluoroscope can be used in the lateral plane (Fig. 79). The usual fluoroscopic table can be used for fluoroscopy in the frontal plane. The intervertebral disks above L2-3 should not be approached transdurally because of the danger of injury to the spinal cord. In the routine study, diskograms are obtained of L3-4, L4-5, and L5-S1.

Markers are placed in the midline between the spinous processes of the vertebrae whose disks are to be injected. These points are marked on the skin with an indelible felt-tip marker. The skin is shaved, scrubbed with povidone-iodine, and draped. The skin beneath the mark is infiltrated with lidocaine. The 20-gauge spinal needle is inserted into the skin and, with the aid of frontal-plane fluoroscopy, is directed downward toward the spinal canal while being maintained in the midline. With the aid of lateral fluoroscopy the depth of the needle and the correct cephalocaudad angulation can be determined so that the needle can be directed toward the intervertebral disk and

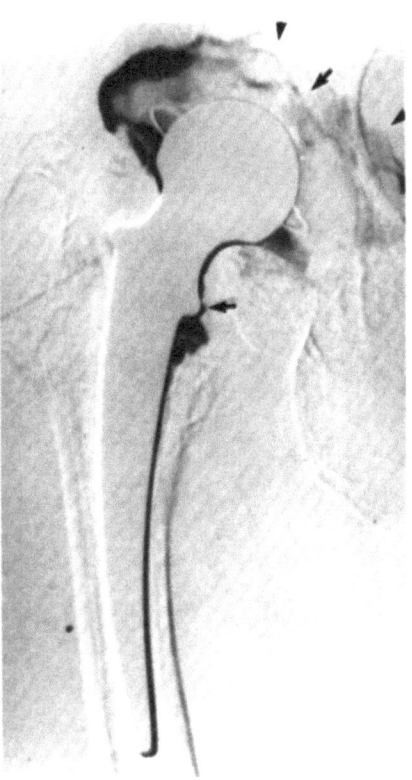

Fig. 72. Subtraction film showing contrast material between the radiopaque cement and the bone (*arrows*), which suggests loosening of the prosthesis. The black area adjacent to the medial aspect of the stem of the femoral component of the prosthesis is artifact due to failure of the scout film and the reversal film to be exactly superimposed.

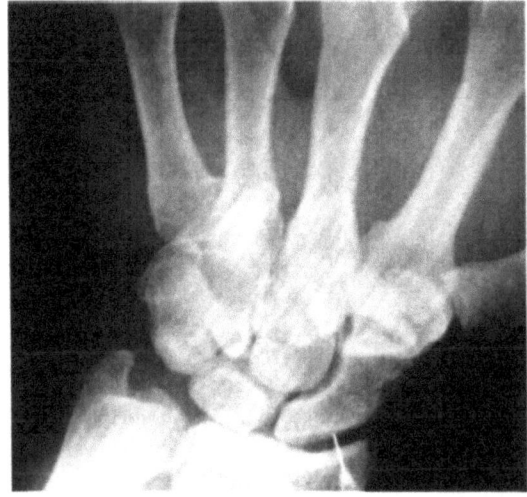

Fig. 73. Joint puncture at the radiocarpal space over the midportion of the navicular bone.

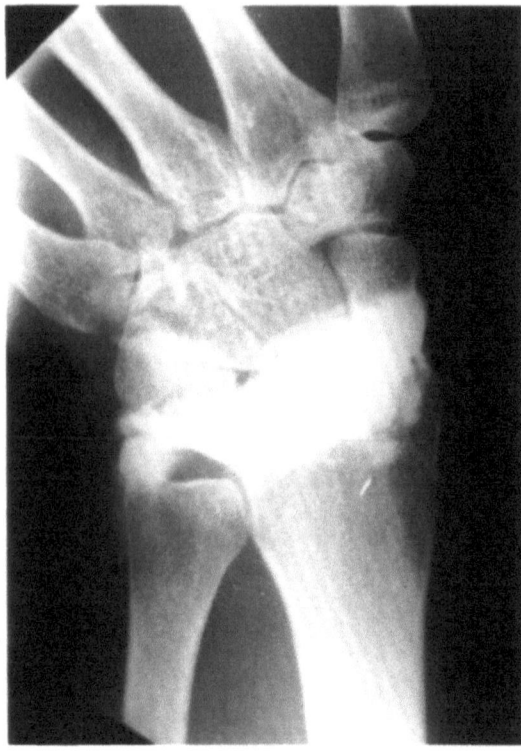

Fig. 74. Arthrogram of normal wrist showing the injected contrast material remaining in the radiocarpal space.

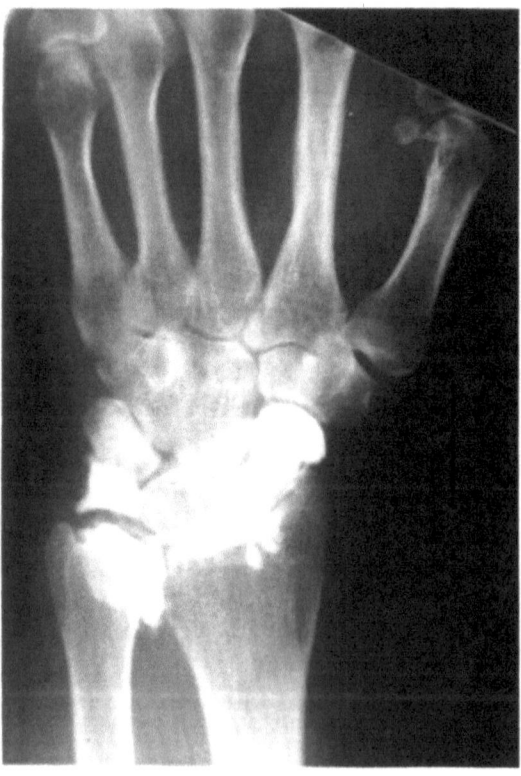

advanced to a level just above the posterior dura.

The 25-gauge spinal needle is then inserted through the 20-gauge needle, and this thin needle is pushed through the posterior dura, subarachnoid space, anterior dura, and into the intervertebral disk (Fig. 80). Mild pain occurs when the needle punctures the anterior dura. A characteristic soft, rubbery sensation is noted when the needle enters the disk. The needle should be able to penetrate the disk easily without resistance. If possible, the needle is placed in the center of the disk and its position observed by frontal- and lateral-plane fluoroscopy.

If the 25-gauge needle cannot be directed into the disk, then it must be removed and the position and angulation of the 20-gauge needle changed. Because of the sharp lordotic angulation at L5-S1, a vertical path of the needle toward the L5-S1 disk space may be impossible, and the 25-gauge needle will tend to strike the inferior aspect of the L-5 vertebral body instead of entering the disk. It often helps to bend the tip of the 25-gauge needle before it is inserted so that it will bend in a caudad direction toward the disk.

It is frequently difficult to adequately visualize the L5-S1 disk space on lateral-plane fluoroscopy with the C arm because of the thickness of the body in this region. Insertion of the needles into the L3-4 and L4-5 intervertebral disks is usually easier. If the exact position and depth of the 25-gauge needle are uncertain on fluoroscopy, then radiographs should be obtained before injection. Ordinary 60% meglumine, sodium diatrizoate, or iothalamate is used for the injection.

Considerable pressure is required to inject a normal intervertebral disk, which can usually accept about 0.5–1 cc of contrast material (Figs. 81 and 82). A 1- or 2-cc syringe should be used for the injection. Contrast material can be extravased through the needle tract if the disk is overdistended. A degenerated disk offers little resistance to injection, and a maxi-

Fig. 75. Contrast material in both the radiocarpal and radioulnar spaces, indicating perforation of the triangular cartilage.

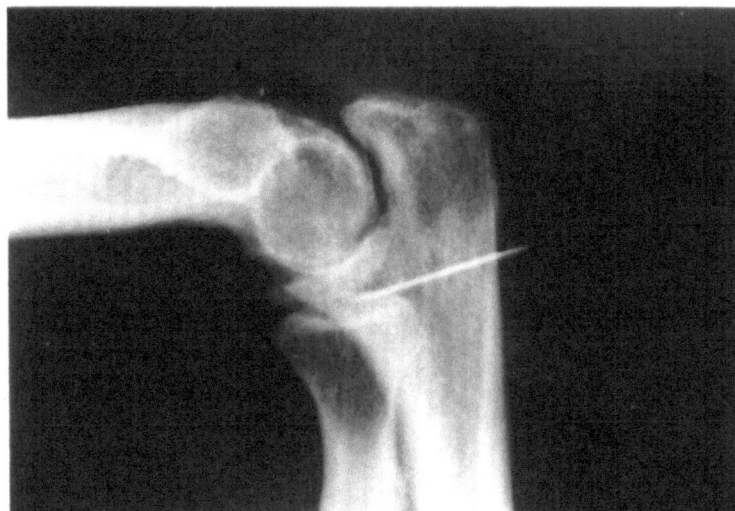

Fig. 76. Fluoroscopic visualization of the proper position of the needle over the radial head with the elbow in the lateral position.

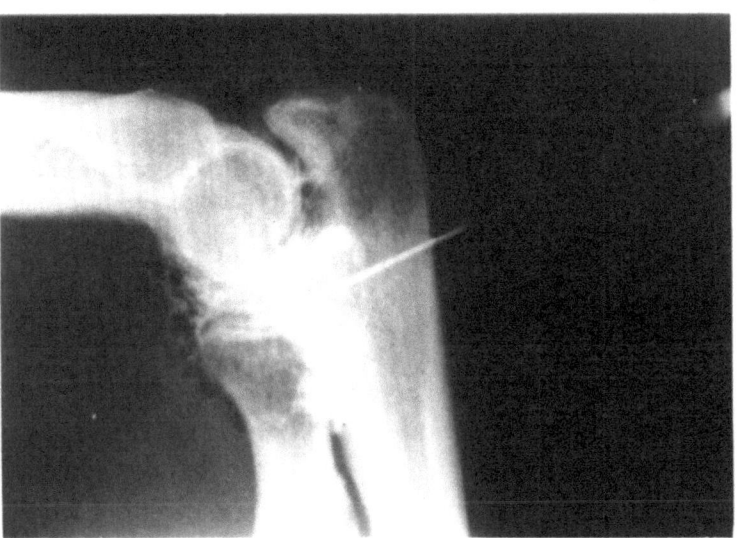

Fig. 77. Injection of contrast material and of air for double-contrast arthrography.

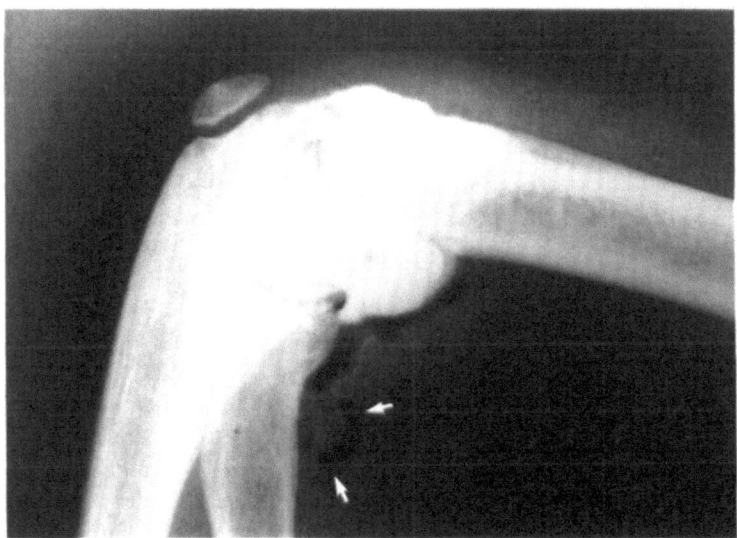

Fig. 78. Loose body within the elbow joint capsule.

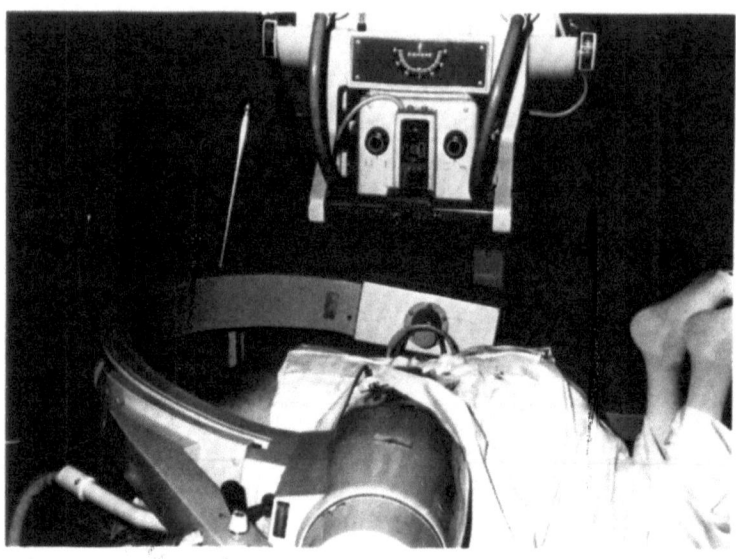

Fig. 79. A portable C-arm fluoroscope for the lateral plane.

mum of 2 cc should be injected. Contrast material that has leaked out of the disk and into the extradural space can irritate the nerve roots and cause severe pain. Stimulation of the patient's pain syndrome by distension of a

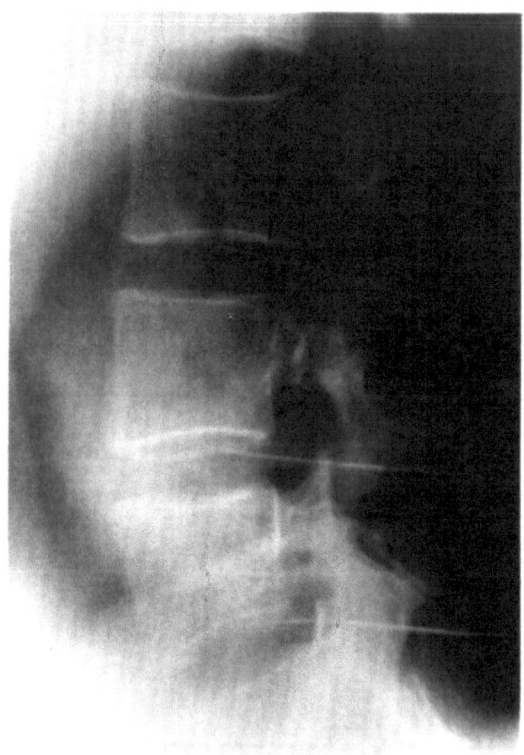

Fig. 80. Insertion of needle into intervertebral disk.

disk has been considered to be evidence of a clinically significant pathologic condition at that level. This sign, however, is difficult to interpret, and the findings are not always reliable. Lidocaine or steroids can be injected into the disks during diskography if requested by the referring physician.

After injection of all three disks, AP and lateral radiographs are obtained with the fluoroscopic units. The 25-gauge and 20-gauge needles are removed together because there is danger that the 25-gauge needle may shear off if it is removed first. AP and lateral films of the spine are obtained with the overhead tube because the technical quality is better than with fluoroscopic spot films. Lateral films of the patient standing and in flexion and extension may help to visualize bulging disks.

Infectious spondylitis is a very rare complication after diskography if a sterile technique has been maintained. The hyperosmolar water-soluble contrast materials, sodium and meglumine diatrizoate and iothalamate, are neurotoxic and can cause severe reactions if injected into the subarachnoid space. Inadvertent subarachnoid and extradural injection should not occur if care is taken to confirm that the needle is in the proper position before injection. The thin 25-gauge needle can break in the patient's back and should be carefully manipulated in positioning and removal. Ordinarily diskography causes more pain and discomfort than myelography; however, usually the procedure is easily tolerated. The patient should remain in the prone or supine position for 24 hours after diskography, just as after myelography.

Percutaneous Needle Biopsy of Bone

Percutaneous needle biopsy of bone can be performed by radiologists. With closed bone biopsy, major surgery to confirm or make the diagnosis of metastatic disease may be avoided. It is valuable in lesions of the vertebral bodies in which radiographic differentiation may be difficult or impossible.

Biopsy sites are located by radiologic examination and radionuclide bone scanning. The most easily approached and safest area for biopsy is chosen. The iliac bone is ideal because it is a superficial non-weight-bearing bone with lesions that usually can easily be seen by fluoroscopy. Biopsy of the spine presents greater potential for complication than biopsy of the pelvic bones.

There are two major types of percutaneous needle biopsy of bone: aspiration and trephine. Aspiration biopsy is less traumatic because smaller needles are used than in trephine biopsy; however, its great disadvantage is the small specimen obtained. Trephine biopsy, in which a core of bone is obtained, has reduced but not completely eliminated this problem. The biopsy specimen may be distorted or damaged, making pathologic interpretation difficult. With sclerotic lesions the bone specimen is often damaged during biopsy. With purely lytic lesions there may be no bone left near the center of the lesion, and the peripheral portions of the lesion may have to be sampled. Skilled and experienced bone pathologists are required to properly interpret the cytologic and pathologic specimens from closed needle biopsy.

Aspiration biopsy is used mainly in suspected infectious spondylitis to obtain fragments of bone and disk material for culture and sensitivity testing. For diagnosis of neoplastic disease, trephine bone biopsy is preferable.

Biplane fluoroscopy makes biopsy of the spine much easier. Lateral radiography can be

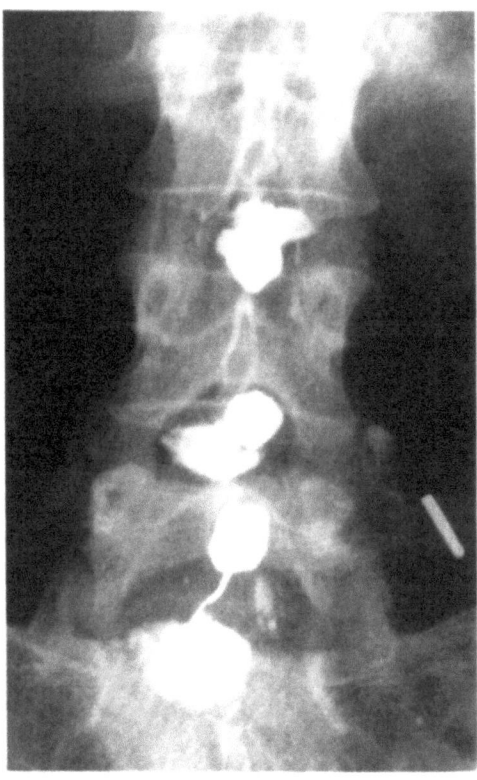

Fig. 81. Needles in the midline with contrast material injected into L3-4, L4-5, and L5-S1 intervertebral disks.

utilized instead of lateral fluoroscopy to localize a needle; however, this becomes tedious and increases the potential risks of the procedure. We use a portable C-arm fluoroscope for lateral-plane fluoroscopy and an ordinary fluoroscopic table for frontal-plane fluoroscopy. For biopsy of the pelvic and long bones use ordinary single-plane image-intensified fluoroscopy.

Anatomy

The anatomy in the region where the biopsy is to be performed should be reviewed in a textbook of anatomy and on a skeleton so that any important structures in the path of the needle can be avoided.

Purpose

To determine if suspected metastatic disease of
    bone is actually present

To differentiate between collapse of vertebral bodies due to osteoporosis and that due to metastatic disease

To diagnose infectious spondylitis and osteomyelitis

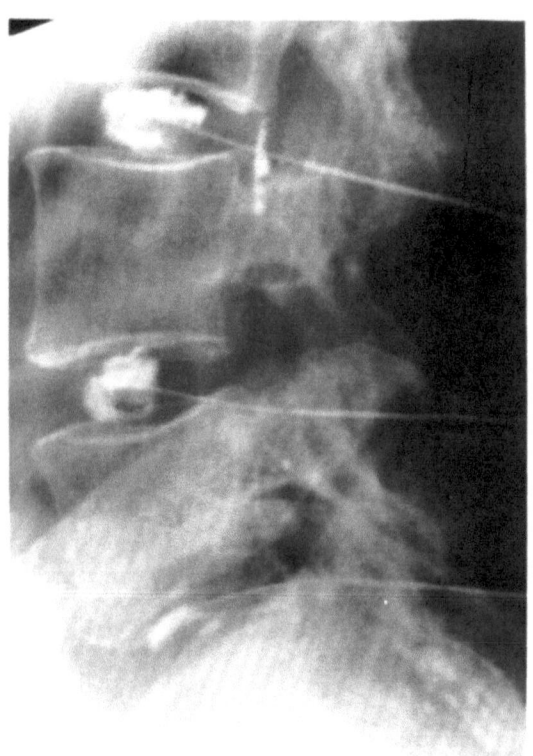

Fig. 82. On the lateral film, contrast material is seen in the intervertebral disks. The 25-gauge needle has been bent so that it curves downward and can enter the center of the L5-S1 disk.

Equipment

Standard (aspiration) biopsy tray (Fig. 83)

Craig needle set (Fig. 84), consisting of (a) a guide with a pointed but not very sharp end, (b) a serrated cutting needle that slides over the cannula, (c) a cannula that can slide over the guide, and (d) a handle that attaches to the needle

18-gauge biopsy needle

Ackerman needle

The Craig needle is the one most often used for trephine bone biopsy.

Technique

The patient is placed on a fluoroscopic table in a position in which the lesion is most easily seen on fluoroscopy and the biopsy site is most easily accessible. With the aid of fluoroscopy the site of the lesion is marked on the skin with an indelible felt-tip marker. This area is scrubbed with povidone-iodine and draped. The skin beneath the mark is infiltrated with lidocaine, and a small incision is made at the site with a scalpel. The 18-gauge needle is inserted and directed toward the lesion with the aid of fluoroscopy while lidocaine is intermittently injected through it into the soft tissues and into the periosteum in the area of the lesion (Fig. 85). The 18-gauge needle is then removed, and the guide of the Craig needle is inserted through the skin incision and directed toward the lesion with the aid of fluoroscopy. When the guide reaches the edge of the lesion the cannula is passed over the guide and pushed

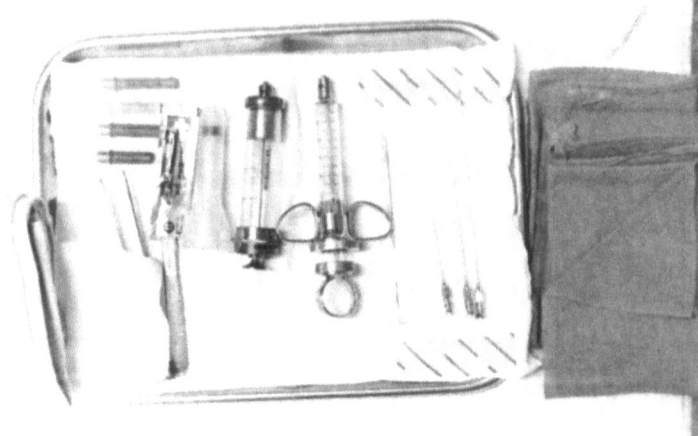

Fig. 83. Standard biopsy tray, which includes the necessary equipment for percutaneous needle biopsy (aspiration).

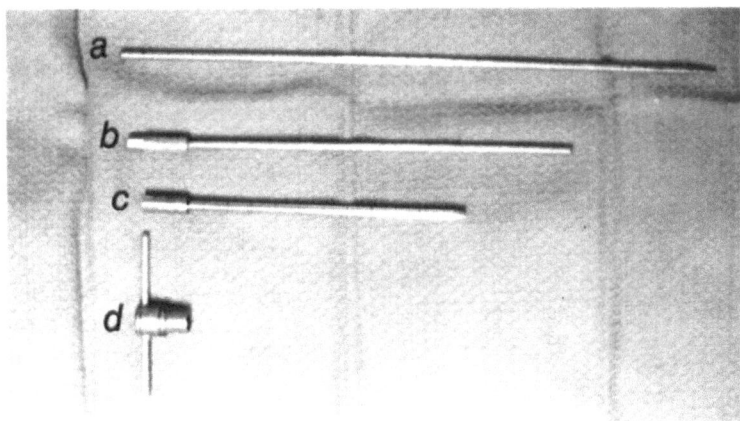

Fig. 84. Important components of the Craig needle biopsy set.

until it meets the cortex adjacent to the bony lesion. The guide is then removed and the serrated cutting needle is passed through the cannula. With the aid of the handle that can be attached and with a twisting motion and pressure, the cutting needle is inserted into the bone (Fig. 86). The cutting needle can extend for a maximum of 2.5 cm past the cannula. It is advisable to take radiographs with the biopsy needle in the lesion so that there will be documentation that the actual area of the lesion was sampled (Fig. 87).

The handle is removed, a syringe is attached to the cutting needle, and suction is applied. The cutting needle is removed, but the cannula remains in place. If the biopsy is successful, there should be a core of bone within the hollow cutting needle. After removal the specimen is placed in a bottle of formalin and sent to the pathology laboratory. Smears are made of soft-tissue material that may have been aspirated into the needle or syringe. Aspirated fluid or soft-tissue material should be placed in a bottle of alcohol and sent to the cytology laboratory.

Needle biopsy of bone may be painful because the periosteum is sensitive. Intramuscular or intravenous administration of meperidine (Demerol) and diazepam (Valium) for premedication is helpful. Often percutaneous needle biopsy can be done on an outpatient basis, but this depends on the site of the lesion and the patient's condition. The patient should be observed for several hours after the biopsy to make certain that hemorrhage has not occurred.

In biopsy of a vertebral body, knowledge of the anatomy is especially important. In the thoracic region the needle should be inserted approximately 4 cm from the midline so that it will pass only through the paravertebral

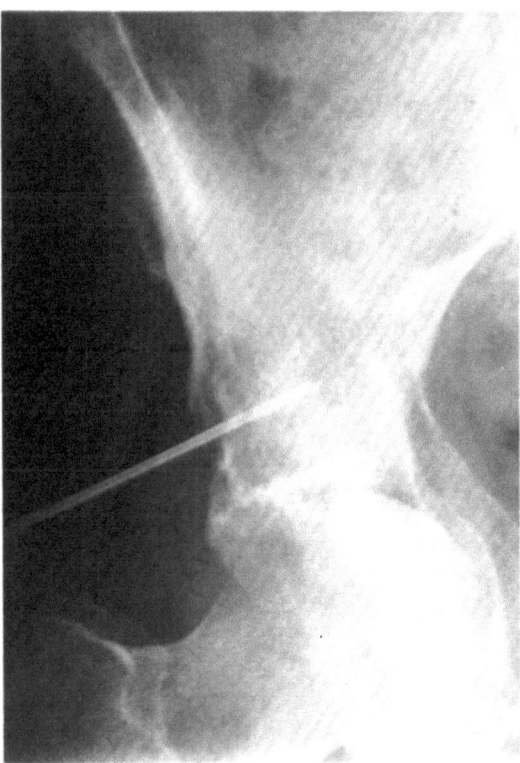

Figure 85. Biopsy needle inserted into the lytic lesion of the iliac bone. The 18-gauge biopsy needle is usually inserted first, both to anesthetize the periosteum and to probe the lesion to ascertain that there will be no damage to a vascular structure that could lead to hemorrhage.

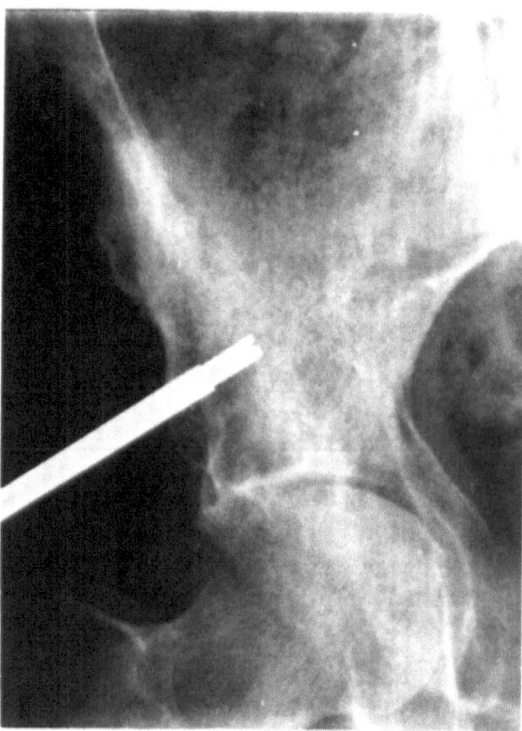

Fig. 86. Craig needle with the serrated edge inserted through the cannula into the lesion.

muscle mass; the more lateral the insertion of the needle the greater the danger of penetration of the pleura and lung. The needle should be inserted somewhat inferior to the vertebral body that is to be entered so that it will pass over the superior portion of the rib below the lesion. The needle often strikes the transverse process, and considerable manipulation may be necessary to get it around this structure so that it can enter the vertebral body. In the spine, as elsewhere, the thin 18-gauge needle should be inserted first to anesthetize the needle tract and bone and to explore the path from the skin to bone. The stylet of the 18-gauge needle should be removed at various intervals and aspiration attempted so that if the needle enters the spinal canal or any vascular structures, fluid or blood will be removed. Very little damage can be done with an 18-gauge needle; however, nerves and blood vessels can be severely damaged with the large trephine bone biopsy needle.

In the lumbar region the needle can be inserted up to 7 cm lateral to the midline and still remain in the paravertebral muscles and avoid the kidneys. This more lateral approach

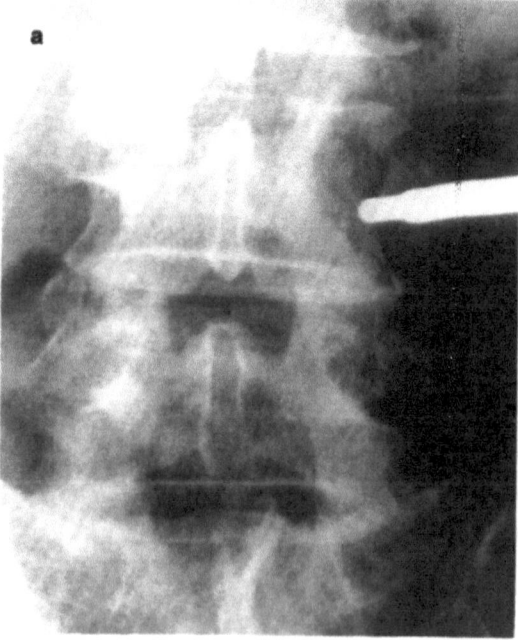

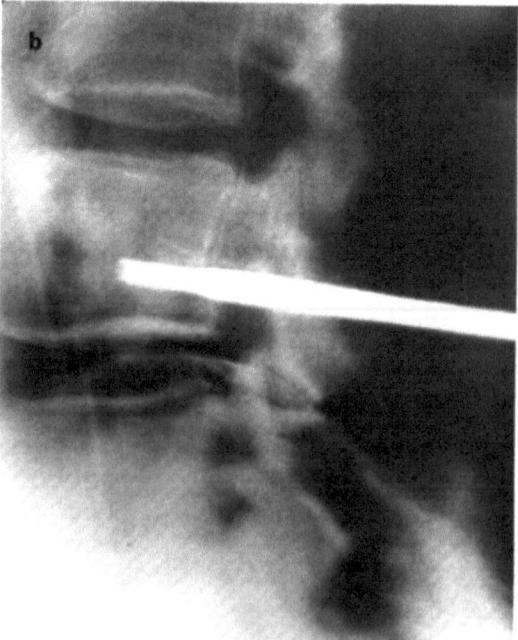

Fig. 87, a and **b.**   Radiographs showing the Craig needle inserted into the destructive lesion of L-4. **a** AP; **b** lateral.

makes it easier to avoid the transverse process and makes biopsy of the lumbar vertebrae easier than that of the thoracic vertebrae. There is less potential risk in biopsy of the lumbar vertebrae because there is no danger of pneumothorax, and there is more free space in the spinal canal in the lumbar region so that any bleeding is less likely to cause compression of the nerves or spinal cord.

Percutaneous needle biopsy of a rib presents some difficulties. Care must be taken that the needle penetrates only the cortical surface of the rib rather than the entire rib and into the lung. Aspiration biopsy of the ribs should be done carefully under fluoroscopic control.

Myelography

With the approval of metrizamide (Amipaque) for general use, a safe water-soluble contrast material has finally replaced the old standard, iophendylate (Pantopaque), as the contrast medium of choice for myelography. In numerous clinical trials, metrizamide has proven its merit and safety. Not only is it easier to use because it does not have to be removed, but it provides superior diagnostic quality. This nonionic liquid allows visualization of nerve roots and root sleeves in all instances (Fig. 88). Although seizures may occasionally occur with its use, they are rare and need not preclude its employment in the majority of patients. Air myelography, utilized rarely in the past, also has been supplanted by myelography with this new contrast agent.

The package inserts supplied with metrizamide are quite specific about preparation of the various concentrations. Generally a volume of 10–15 cc is desirable for either lumbar or cervical studies. Concentrations, however, vary from 170–180 mg/ml for lumbar examination to 250–300 mg/ml for cervical examination. The higher concentration in the latter takes into account the dilution that will occur as the contrast medium is manipulated from the lumbar to cervical region.

Equipment

20- or 22-gauge needle

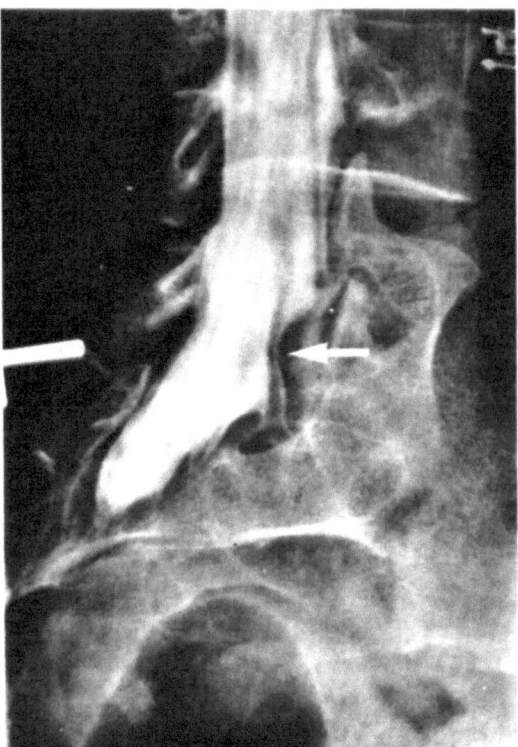

Fig. 88. Oblique myelogram, obtained after injection of metrizamide, demonstrating extrinsic impression of L5-S1 nerve roots.

Patient Positioning

Semi-upright (for injection)
Prone oblique

The prone oblique position is used to keep the bolus of contrast material concentrated as it goes from the lumbar to cervical region and to minimize its breakup as it passes over the thoracic kyphosis.

Filming

Fluoroscopic spot films
Overhead radiographs

Since the needle is removed once the contrast agent is injected there is much more freedom of maneuverability during filming. Although both the spot films and the radiographs are suitable for imaging of any area, for ease of patient handling and control the former are preferred.

Position

Cross-table lateral views
Lateral decubitus views

Technique (by Means of Lumbar Puncture)

Both lumbar and cervical studies can be performed by means of injection at L2-3 or L3-4. Fluoroscopic control of the needle puncture, although requiring a few more minutes, will insure both proper disk space and midline needle placement. Proper midline needle placement is not as critical when metrizamide is employed as it was when iophendylate, which must be removed at the end of the study, was used. After the skin is marked under fluoroscopic control it is cleansed and dermal local anesthesia induced. Deeper anesthesia is not necessary as long as a midline puncture route is followed.

The needle is slowly advanced, fluoroscopic views being occasionally obtained to insure proper alignment. (Although an 18-gauge needle was standard with use of iophendylate, a 20- or even 22-gauge needle may be used with the less viscous metrizamide.) A distinct dural "pop" is usually felt even with the smaller-gauge needles, and after the initial flow of fluid is seen following the pop, the needle is carefully advanced 2–3 mm and then rotated before fluid is removed for laboratory analysis. This last maneuver should insure that the entire bevel of the needle is in a subarachnoid position. Fluoroscopic visualization of injection of iophendylate (Pantopaque) in a semi-upright patient would show subarachnoid placement because the oily material breaks up into droplets that quickly fall caudally. Metrizamide does not form such characteristic droplets, and fluoroscopic control of injection is not necessary.

Differences in injection technique are, however, important. Metrizamide has a higher specific gravity than cerebrospinal fluid and it is desirable to minimize mixing the two. To this end, metrizamide should be injected as slowly as possible with the patient in the semi-upright position. This will concentrate the contrast agent in the caudal sac, minimizing its dilution and therefore maintaining its radio-opacity longer. Eventually, however, the material will become less opaque as it is gradually diluted and reabsorbed. Table tilting should be slow and steady to preserve the bolus of contrast medium as much as possible. Of course, once the injection is complete, the needle may be removed.

Technique (by Means of Suboccipital Puncture)

This technique should be used whenever the lumbar puncture does not yield satisfactory results. The back of the head is shaved, and the position of the dura is ascertained between the base of the skull and C-1 posteriorly. The needle is then advanced under fluoroscopic control until it strikes the posterior aspect of the occipital bone. It is withdrawn slightly and "walked" down the occipital bone until the occipital C-1 membrane is punctured. There is a relatively large space anterior to the membrane into which the needle can be placed. Once fluid is obtained the contrast material can be injected at this level and the needle removed. It is unwise to manipulate the head or neck while the needle is in place at this level. In a patient with possible tonsillar herniation or arteriovenous malformations the puncture can be made somewhat lower, at the C-2 level, where a lateral or posterior approach can be used, although the former is somewhat easier and safer.

Complications

Headache
Nausea and vomiting
Seizures

Postprocedure Care

Postmyelographic care of the patient remains the same as after use of iophendylate. The occurrence of "minor" complications (headache, etc.) is perhaps, more frequent with the newer contrast agent than with the oily material. Although rare, seizures do occur and may be delayed in presentation. Thus measures to combat them, at least a tongue blade beside the bed, would be wise for several hours following the study.

Percutaneous Transhepatic Cholangiography

Increasing use of the percutaneous approach in evaluation of the biliary tree has been spurred by reports of great success with the Chiba University or "skinny" needle method. Whether or not this needle is responsible for increasing success of this examination is not clear, but it has had some effect. At institutions in which endoscopic retrograde cannulation of the common duct is accomplished with ease, transhepatic cholangiography by retrograde injection may be of value in further evaluation of complete obstruction. Percutaneous transhepatic cholangiography may generally be completed within 30 minutes and may offer potential therapeutic benefits in obstructive lesions in which percutaneous catheter placement may provide drainage.

In the past these examinations were scheduled as preoperative studies, but we perform them as any other diagnostic special procedure. Although considerable attention has been recently given to the skinny needle approach, the success of this needle may, more likely, rest in the technique of injecting contrast material while withdrawing the needle rather than aspirating to confirm its presence in the biliary tree. If a patient has obvious high-grade obstructive jaundice and a drainage procedure is considered, a sheath-needle apparatus may be used; if a medical-surgical jaundice diagnostic problem is encountered, then the thin-walled needle is used initially. The techniques are similar regardless of which needle is used.

Purpose

To evaluate the intrahepatic biliary tree
To evaluate and decompress complete obstruction of the common bile duct

Equipment

18- and 19-gauge sheath-needle assemblies
22- and 23-gauge thin-walled needles

Patient Positioning

Supine (anterior or lateral approach)

Technique by Means of Anterior Approach

The objective of needle placement is puncture of the anterior surface of the liver and needle passage through the major segmental ducts where they converge toward the hilum, while at the same time strictly avoiding puncture of extrahepatic structures, particularly the gallbladder and vessels of the porta hepatis. The ideal needle tract provides sufficient hepatic parenchyma to tamponade large vessels or ducts punctured by the needle. The anterior approach generally involves directing the needle more centrally in the liver.

The patient is placed on the fluoroscopy table. The skin surface is marked over the diaphragm during deep inspiration. Air may be injected through a nasogastric tube or via ingested soda, and the duodenal bulb is marked during inspiration. This is the entry site of the needle through the skin. The direction of the needle is planned from all available anatomic information: fluoroscopy, previous gastrointestinal studies, liver scans, direct observation, palpation, etc. In general, the needle is angulated cranially from 15° to 45°, the angle increasing with greater distance between the duodenal bulb and diaphragm, and 0° to 30° toward the patient's right side. These angles will vary according to the size and shape of the liver. Depth of insertion varies from 4–7 in.

After induction of local anesthesia and infiltration along the projected needle tract to the peritoneum, a small skin incision is made to facilitate needle passage. The needle-sheath assembly is then passed to the peritoneum. During suspended respiration the needle is inserted as planned and the inner stylet quickly removed. Normal respiration is resumed (by patient and operator), and a short length of flexible tubing and a syringe with contrast material diluted to 30%–50% are attached to the catheter.

Small amounts of contrast medium are injected initially, while the catheter or needle is slowly withdrawn. This contrast material may be deposited interstitially, or quickly flow through hepatic or portal vein branches, or fill bile ducts. When bile ducts fill, additional contrast medium is injected until a diagnostic cholangiogram is obtained. Bile is withdrawn when it can be easily aspirated, usually when ducts are quite dilated, but priority is given to obtaining a satisfactory cholangiogram. Many examinations are successful despite inability to aspirate bile. This has been true in all patients with nonobstructive jaundice.

If the initial puncture fails to effect visualization of bile ducts, additional attempts are made, the number depending on patient tolerance and the "quality" of the punctures. (Quality refers to the needle tract location in the liver.)

Often radiologists have attempted to direct the needle in a different direction from the initial puncture site. Repeated punctures may result in the needle being placed in a path almost identical to the previous passes. For this reason, if attempts are unsuccessful, choosing another skin site or changing to a lateral approach might be helpful.

Technique by Means of Lateral Approach

As in the anterior approach, knowledge of the anatomy of the liver in a given patient is of considerable value in completing successful studies. In a patient with cirrhosis, in whom the right lobe is small and the left lobe prominent, the entry site will be different from that in a patient in whom the right lobe is prominent. The latter is the technically easier to approach.

Landmarks to be indicated on the skin surface are the costophrenic angle, during deep inspiration; the dome of the diaphragm; and the anticipated placement site of the needle.

The entry site is located 2–3 cm anterior to the midaxillary line and at the 10th through 12th interspace, depending on the patient's anatomy. The ideal needle path would be horizontal; however, this may not be possible because of the patient's anatomy.

Under fluoroscopy the thick central portion of the right lobe of the liver is marked on the skin of the anterior abdominal wall. This mark is extremely helpful because it provides an imaginary straight line from the entry site on the skin to the point in the right lobe to which the needle is being directed.

After placement of the needle deep into the liver substance a Venotube with dilute contrast agent is attached to it, and small amounts of the medium are injected as the needle is slowly withdrawn. Once the position of the needle in the biliary tree is confirmed, contrast material is continuously injected until an adequate cholangiogram is obtained.

With the injection technique, one may obtain visualization of the hepatic vein, portal vein, and hepatic lymphatics (Fig. 89). In patients in whom cirrhosis is suspected, measurement of portal pressure should be considered if the portal venous system is entered during cholangiography. This will often provide adjunctive information concerning morphologic aspects of the biliary tree.

The success of these percutaneous techniques of cholangiography is clearly due to the withdrawal-intermittent injection procedure, and this may contribute to safety by reducing the number of needle punctures. The biliary tree is often filled through small, relatively peripheral, sometimes unidentifiable, branches even when there is gross ductal dilatation. The catheter tip is not actually in the bile ducts for many cholangiograms, and small ducts that may have been punctured fill via the needle tract or interstitial deposit.

In our hands, percutaneous transhepatic cholangiography has been successful in 90%–99% of cases of obstructive lesions (Fig. 90). In nonobstructive lesions, the procedure has been successful in 80%–90% of cases.

Complications

Cholangitis

In patients with partially obstructing lesions this has been the most important complication of the procedure. Although it can be managed with antibiotic therapy, we regard cholangiographic evidence of cholangitis, e.g., demonstration of small liver abscesses communicating with bile ducts, as an emergency situation and recommend immediate operation.

Bile peritonitis

Although this has been reported as a complication, in the past it was the indication for preoperative use of the procedure. Serious bile peritonitis has not occurred as a complication in our series of more than 250 studies, although occurrence of localized, self-limited peritonitis may occur related to small bile leaks.

Subcapsular hemorrhage

This may occur especially in patients who are poorly cooperative or tachypneic during the procedure.

Free peritoneal bleeding

This represents a potential complication in our series. It may occur especially in patients with poor coagulation factors.

Pain

Right upper-quadrant and subscapular pain may occur with subcapsular injection of contrast medium. It is usually transient and relieved with parenterally administered analgesia. Epigastric pain may be present as well.

Occasionally a patient experiences severe pain on injection of contrast material into obstructed bile ducts, most commonly when obstruction is due to calculi, as opposed to chronic obstruction. When marked obstruction of the biliary tree is encountered, aspiration of the biliary tree should be attempted to avoid dramatically increasing the biliary pressure when contrast medium is injected.

Preprocedure and Postprocedure Care

Administration of broad-spectrum antibiotics is usually started 24 hours prior to the procedure and continued for several days following it in patients with high degrees of obstruction or undergoing drainage procedures.

Percutaneous Drainage of the Biliary Tree

As an adjunct to percutaneous cholangiography the biliary tree may be temporarily or permanently decompressed by the placement of larger indwelling catheters. In patients with carcinoma of the pancreas or other common bile duct strictures, biliary stents may be placed providing relief of jaundice, as well as restoring the flow of bile toward the duodenum.

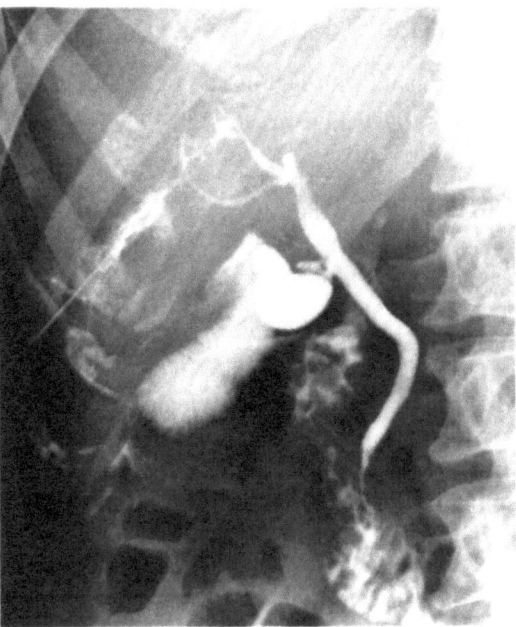

Fig. 89. Skinny-needle cholangiogram in a patient with cholestatic jaundice showing normal biliary tree. Some interstitial contrast is noted, and good filling of the common bile duct and gallbladder is accomplished, yet the specific biliary radicle puncture cannot be easily identified.

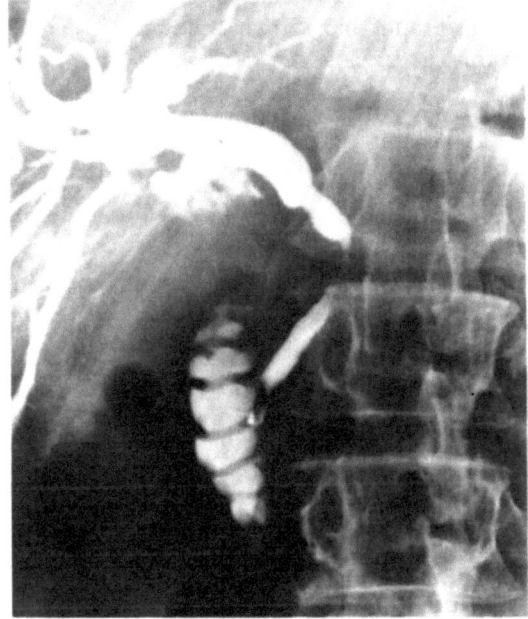

Fig. 90. Carcinoma of the pancreas demonstrated by percutaneous transhepatic choliangiography.

Technique

In patients with high-grade obstruction documented biochemically, intravenous antibiotics are initiated prior to intervention.

A polyethylene sheath apparatus is used for initial entry into the biliary tree. A more central puncture of the biliary tree is recommended, with a horizontal needle course. Once bile is aspirated, a guide wire is passed into the distal biliary tree. At this point the polyethylene sheath may be passed over the guide wire and additional cholangiography performed. Alternatively, an 8.3 F specially designed "pigtail" catheter may be placed for drainage. Once the stricture is traversed by the guide wire, the wire is further passed through the ampulla of Vater into the duodenum. The end of the catheter is further advanced into the duodenum for permanent drainage.

Once desired catheter position is achieved, the catheter is secured to the skin surface with sutures. Generally, initial drainage is external for 24–48 hours to establish flow during the acute postprocedure period. The tube may then be closed with a stopcock and covered with a dressing.

As an adjunct, collection of bile from the vicinity of the tumor may often result in positive cytologic diagnosis. If negative, percutaneous aspiration biopsy may follow for obtaining histologic diagnosis.

Splenoportography

Purpose

To investigate symptoms of portal hypertension or stasis:
   Cirrhosis
   Cruveilhier-Baumgarten syndrome (cirrhosis with patency of umb. vein)
   Budd-Chiari syndrome (obs. or occl. hepatic veins)
   Congenital stenosis and cavernous transformation of portal vein
   Acquired stenosis of portal vein
   Portal phlebitis
To investigate unexplained gastrointestinal hemorrhage

To investigate symptoms involving suprameso-colic viscera:
   Neoplasms and chronic inflammation of pancreas
   Celiac lymphadenopathy
   Primary and secondary tumors of liver
   Hepatic cysts or other space-occupying lesions

Contraindications

Significant disturbance of blood-coagulation mechanism
Intrasplenic collections (cyst, tumors, abscess)
Large amount of ascites (floating spleen)

Equipment

Metallic skin marker
Short flexible-rubber tube
Three-way stopcock
25-cm connector tube
Water manometer
10-cc and 20-cc syringes
Lidocaine (Xylocaine) 1%
No. 25 and 22 needles for anesthesia

Patient Positioning

Supine

Injection

60 cc diatrizoate meglumine and diatrizoate sodium (Renografin-76) 8 cc/s

Note: At the end of the injection (as the film is being exposed) the needle is removed with a fast movement during apnea.

Film Sequence

Central beam—2 fingerbreadths below xiphoid process

15–20 films: 2-s delay
1 film/s for 13 s; 1/3 s to run out
Total filming 27–33 s

Technique

In preparation for the procedure the patient is permitted nothing by mouth. A complete blood work-up is done, including baseline hematocrit determination.

It is extremely important to explain and rehearse the procedure with the patient. The patient is told to stop breathing (voluntary apnea) anytime this is requested (preferably in midexpiration) and to resume breathing quietly, without taking a deep breath. The patient is told to refrain from talking, coughing, and making sudden movements during the procedure.

Fluoroscopy is performed to locate the spleen and to select the puncture site. During voluntary apnea in midexpiration the position of the spleen (splenic shadow, stomach, colonic flexure) is noted and the splenic hilum identified. The metallic marker is placed on the anterior chest wall at the location of the splenic hilum (after some experience is gained this can be omitted). During voluntary apnea the puncture site is selected. It should be below the lowest insertion of the diaphragm and at the point where the spleen is closest to the abdominal wall. A small needle is placed at the selected puncture site and the site rechecked. This point is usually at the level of the ninth or tenth intercostal space in the posterior axillary line (normal spleen) or the midaxillary line (splenomegaly). The skin over the puncture area is prepared and the patient is draped.

Note: Sterile sheets should be on the table close to the left side of the patient.

The skin is anesthetized with lidocaine (Xylocaine) 1%.

For the puncture the needle is directed cranially and in the frontal plane toward a spot 2–3 cm from the hilar mark. The skin is penetrated and the needle advanced until the rough surface of the spleen is felt. During apnea the spleen is rapidly penetrated (2–3 cm in a normal spleen and 3–5 cm in an enlarged spleen). If blood returns through the needle during quiet respiration the short tube and stopcock are attached during apnea. Then during quiet respiration the water manometer and a 20-cc syringe containing saline are connected.

The tube is cleaned with saline, and the water manometer is filled with saline. The stopcock is changed so the manometer connects to the short tube (syringe excluded). The splenic pulp pressure is measured once, then three more times.

A test dose of a few cubic centimeters of Renografin-76 is administered during quiet respiration. If the splenic veins are visualized, filming is carried out. If the splenic veins are not visualized at the test injection the needle is slightly advanced or withdrawn during apnea, and another test dose is injected. If the veins are still not visualized, the needle is removed, and another puncture is made with the same technique but no closer than 2 cm to the initial puncture site.

Note: No more than two punctures should be made.

Postprocedure Care

Patient should lie on the left side for 3–4 hours. Hematocrit is determined twice at 4-hour intervals and once the following morning. If there is any subcapsular deposition of contrast agent the patient should be warned of probable discomfort and pain in the left shoulder, and analgesia should be ordered.

Sialography

Purpose

To show parotid gland in relation to adjacent structures
To determine presence of stones and strictures
To detect salivary fistulas
To determine if a mass lesion is intraglandular or extraglandular
To aid in planning an operative procedure
To differentiate lateral nasopharyngeal masses

Contraindications

Acute parotitis (mumps)
Suppurative parotitis

Equipment

Graded silver lacrimal probes
Preferably a 4–5 F catheter and thin-walled Teflon tube, tapered so that the outer diameter of the tip is about 0.5–1 mm (Cook

Incorporated); or no. 14–18 soft plastic intravenous catheter

Rabinov catheter (Cook Incorporated), which has a metallic tip that precludes the need for prior dilatation

Two-way stopcock

Note: Any technique that does not use a closed system, i.e., a catheter, is of questionable value.

Patient Positioning

Seated

Filming

Scout and spot films

Position

AP
Lateral with chin tilted 15° cephalad
Oblique
Submandibular gland; occlusal view

Technique

After the patient is positioned and keeping the tip of the tongue against the soft palate, the duct opening is located: the parotid gland lies against the second molar; the submandibular gland is in the floor of mouth lateral to the frenulum. The area is dried with a cotton sponge or air. The radiologist presses on the gland and looks for a drop of saliva. Once the opening is located it can be dilated with lacrimal probes.

The catheter is connected to the stopcock and to a 2-cc syringe filled with contrast medium. The contrast agent used, depending on specific indication, is iophendylate (Pantopaque) 30%; iodized oil (Lipiodol) 40%; ethiodized oil (Ethiodol) or diatrizoate meglumine and diatrizoate (Renografin-60), which is water soluble. The system is flushed with the medium. The catheter is introduced 1–2 cm within the duct and fastened to the corner of the mouth with a strip of adhesive tape. From this point the examination consists of three phases:

1) Filling phase. Under fluoroscopic control the ducts are gradually filled while multiple spot films (well coned) are obtained in different stages of filling.

Note: Any technique in which the gland is filled blindly should be avoided because subtle duct disease might be missed.

Usually after 1–1.5 cc contrast agent is injected, parenchymal opacification begins; it is marked by a fluffy, cloudy appearance. This terminates the first stage.

2) Parenchymal phase. The stopcock is closed and the syringe removed. Overhead radiograms are obtained: AP, lateral, oblique, and occlusal views.

Note: Any examination limited to the duct system is incomplete, and thus of no value, because filling defects in the gland will be missed. Films are checked for adequacy.

3) Postevacuation phase. The catheter is removed. The patient is given a slice of lemon or a few drops of lemon extract to stimulate salivary secretion; after 10 minutes a lateral view is obtained to determine the degree of evacuation.

Nasopharnyngography

Purpose

To detect small mass lesions within nasopharynx
To detect choanal atresia

Catheters

Rubber or polyethylene (6–8 F)

Patient Positioning

Supine with head dependent. Shoulders elevated so orbitomeatal line is at a 45° angle with the horizontal.

Injection

10–20 ml into each nostril

Position

Scout films:
AP with vertical beam
Lateral cross-table (tube at 40 in.)
AP vertical
Lateral cross-table
Submentovertex with tube 15° cephalad
Submentovertex with tube 30° cephalad
AP erect or standing
Lateral after contrast medium is expelled
AP erect
Lateral erect

Technique

The patient is warned that there will be a sensation of wetness and filling of the nostrils and is instructed to breathe only through the mouth. Premedication and anesthesia are not used. If there is nasal irritation a topical spray is used. A catheter is introduced into each nostril, and contrast material is injected into each.

Bronchography

Purpose

To determine cause of hemoptysis when bronchoscopic findings are normal
To investigate repeated episodes of pneumonia, particularly if the same lobe or lobes are involved
To investigate localized "emphysema" accompanied by wheeze in the same area
To investigate unilateral hilar adenopathy, with or without associated pulmonary lesion, in an adult
To evaluate persistent unilateral pulmonary infiltration not responding to medical therapy
To differentiate persistent cavities and cysts
To evaluate known or suspected congenital anomalies of the bronchial tree

Contraindications

Severe and recent hemoptysis
Significant impairment of pulmonary function, particularly obstructive (In this case probably the wisest procedure is a selective study restricted to the lobe in which disease is suspected.)
Congestive heart failure
Acute pneumonia
Sensitivity to iodine
Acute asthma

Equipment

15-gauge needle with 45° angle
2-cc, 10-cc, and 20-cc syringes
Guide wires 40 cm long, P.E. 116 metallic spring wire with flexible tip
Red KIFA catheter 30 cm long with end-hole and two side-holes in the tapered end
7 F C-3 cobra catheter

Note: The same catheter type, specifically shaped by immersion in hot water is used for selective bronchography.

For apical segments a curve of at least 180° is necessary
For anterior and posterior upper lobe segments the same curve is required but with the addition of a short secondary curve anteriorly or posteriorly.
For the middle lobe and lingula a 90° curve is sufficient.
For lower lobe segments a 30° curve or less is adequate.
Preshaped visceral catheter, in conjunction with a deflector system
Luer-Lok and a two-way adapter
No. 11 blade
Foam-rubber pad

Patient Positioning

For anesthesia and catheter placement: supine with shoulders elevated by the foam-rubber pad and neck hyperextended
For bronchography: lateral decubitus, posterior oblique
For selective bronchography so bronchi will be parallel with the film)
Right upper olbe: right posterior oblique with the left chest elevated 22°
Right middle lobe: right posterior oblique with the left chest elevated 72°
Right lower lobe: right lateral with the pelvis elevated so that the body is at an angle of 25° with the table

Left lower lobe: left lateral with same pelvic elevation as for right lower lobe

Left upper lobe: left posterior oblique 45°

Injection

For unilateral bronchography: 15 ml
Never more than 20 ml

Note: Overfilling of the bronchial tree with contrast medium is one of the most common causes of technically poor studies.

Position

Scout films:
AP
Lateral
Posterior oblique (of the side to be studied)
Spot films:
Lateral decubitus
Posterior oblique
Overhead films (single bolus technique):
Lateral decubitus
Posterior oblique
AP
Overhead films (fractionated-injection technique):
AP
Oblique
Lateral
Delayed erect

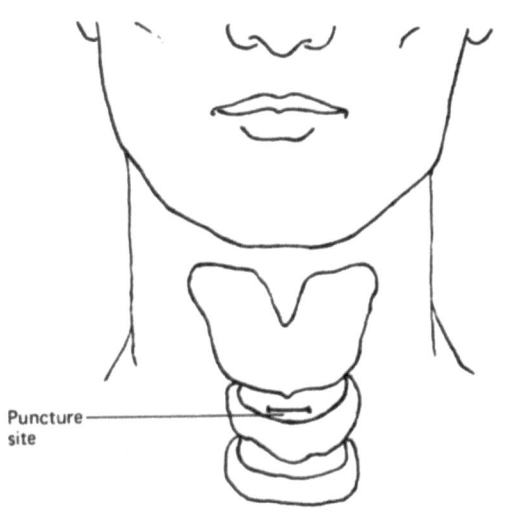

Fig. 91. Anatomic landmarks for transtracheal bronchography.

Technique

It is desirable to know the status of pulmonary function, especially the results of ventilatory tests, since bronchography results in temporary diminution of pulmonary function. Explanation of the procedure to the patient and reassurance are of paramount importance and often make the difference between a good and poor study. The patient is permitted nothing by mouth for 5 hours before the procedure. If bronchiectasis is suspected or if copious sputum is produced, postural drainage is indicated.

Premedication is administered to provide mild sedation, to suppress the cough reflex, and to reduce secretions: codeine phosphate 30–40 mg, secobarbital 50–100 mg, and atropine sulfate 0.4–0.6 mg subcutaneously, are given 1 hour before study.

Barium sulfate suspension seems to be the ideal contrast medium for bronchography, but it is not approved for use in the United States. Oily propyliodine (Dionosil) is usually employed.

The contrast agent should be at room temperature or slightly above. If it is heated, viscosity is reduced and "alveolarization" readily occurs. The contrast medium must be thoroughly shaken to insure even mixing. If desired, viscosity can be increased by pouring off some of the supernatant oil before shaking.

The skin over the cricothyroid membrane is prepared. The cricothyroid membrane is palpated, and the notch between the lower border of the thyroid cartilage and the upper border of the cricoid cartilage is located (Fig. 91). The larynx is firmly grasped between the thumb and the forefinger of the left hand. A no. 25 needle is used to administer 1% lidocaine (Xylocaine) for anesthesia. The area down to and including the cricothyroid membrane is infiltrated with 1–2 ml lidocaine. With a 21-gauge needle the trachea is penetrated through the cricothyroid membrane. Air should be aspirated to ascertain that the trachea has been entered. The table is then tilted into a 10° Trendelenburg position and 1–2 ml lidocaine 1% is injected.

Next the table is tilted 40° above the horizontal. The patient is warned that the next injection will produce cough; 2–3 ml lidocaine is injected forcefully and rapidly, the needle removed very quickly, and the patient allowed to cough. The table is returned to the horizontal position. A stab wound is made in the skin overlying the cricothyroid area with the no. 11 blade. The larynx is grasped firmly and the trachea punctured with a 16-gauge short-bevel needle or Seldinger type of needle. Aspiration of air through this needle gives assurance of proper positioning of its tip. A 16-gauge needle with 45° angle may also be used.

Note: In order to avoid puncture of the posterior wall of the trachea, the index finger is used as a limiting guard, holding the needle approximately 1 cm from the tip and maintaining it at a 45° angle pointing caudally.

A guide wire is introduced through the needle and advanced until its flexible tip is entirely free within the lumen of the trachea. The needle is removed, and the selected catheter is slipped over the wire into the trachea, with the tip within the lower trachea. An additional 2 ml lidocaine is injected here. The pad is removed from beneath the patient's shoulders and placed beneath the head (slight flexion of the head will prevent reflux into the larynx). The catheter is advanced in a main bronchus and placed distal to the upper-lobe bronchus. The patient is turned into a decubitus position with the catheterized side down. The patient is told to exhale; 5 ml lidocaine is injected, following which air is injected to remove all of the anesthetic from the catheter. The patient inhales deeply to disperse the anesthetic through the bronchial tree. The catheter is placed in the main bronchus on the opposite side and the maneuver is repeated. Even in unilateral bronchography both sides should be anesthetized to reduce the chance of coughing.

Note: The maximum amount of anesthetic for an average patient is 300 mg.

Lateral Decubitus with a Single Bolus. With the patient in the lateral decubitus position all orifices of the bronchial tree are dependent and can be filled simultaneously. The catheter is placed in the main bronchus of the side to be examined slightly distal to the upper-lobe

bronchus. The patient is turned in the corresponding lateral decubitus position (the side to be examined down). As a final test for correct anesthesia the patient is instructed to exhale and an additional 1–2 ml lidocaine is injected. The patient is then told to inhale. This should no longer produce cough.

The syringe containing the contrast medium is connected, and the patient instructed to exhale forcefully and not to breathe (Fig. 92). Under fluoroscopic control a bolus of contrast material is rapidly injected. Usually, since the size of the bronchial tree diminishes during exhalation, 7–15 cc contrast material is adequate to fill the major radicles, which are outlined as a solid cast. A spot film is obtained while the patient is in the lateral decubitus position. The patient is instructed to breathe normally which results in further peripheral aspiration of the contrast medium and double-contrast visualization of the bronchi. One more spot film is obtained while the patient is in this position and one spot film is obtained while the patient is in the posterior oblique position.

Note: The patient is not turned to the supine position because there may be spillover to the opposite side.

The patient is again turned to the lateral decubitus position and overhead radiographs taken in the following sequence: (1) lateral decubitus, (2) posterior oblique, (3) AP (in this view some spillover will occur but does not interfere with the visualization of examined side. If considered necessary additional spot films can be taken now.

If the films are satisfactory, the catheter is removed and the patient instructed to breathe deeply and cough vigorously. Any time the patient coughs he or she should press the fingers on the area of puncture to avoid development of subcutaneous emphysema. A delayed (15–30 minutes) erect film is obtained.

This technique has several advantages. It is simple and rapid. It is convenient for the patient, who does not have to roll into various positions. There is no spillover into the contralateral side except during filming of the last AP radiogram when it is not objectionable.

Positional, Fractionated Injection. An aver-

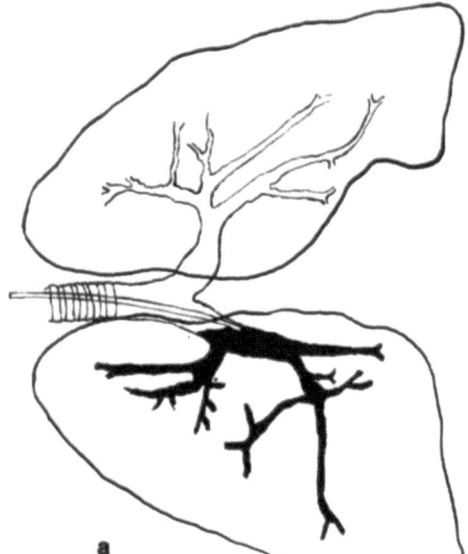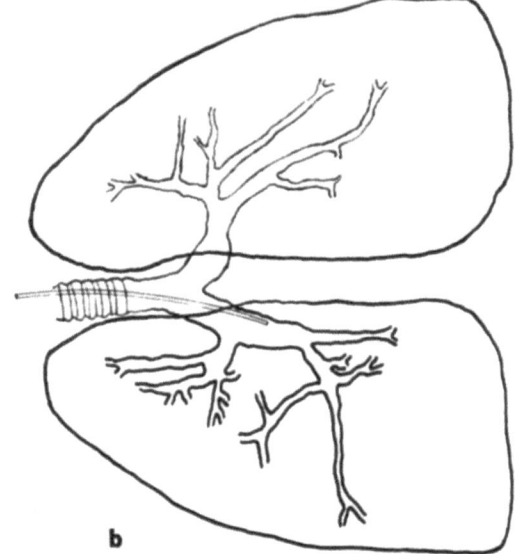

Fig. 92, a and b. Decubitus injection of contrast medium for unilateral bronchography (after Amplatz). **a** Injection of contrast material in the right lateral decubitus position results in optimal filling of the dependent bronchi. **b** An optimal bronchogram is produced after inspiration.

age of 15–20 cc contrast agent is injected into each main bronchus as the patient is placed in different positions; spot films are exposed when the segmental bronchi of each lobe are well filled.

The tip of the catheter is advanced into the main bronchus of the side to be examined. The table is tilted so that the patient's head is 15°–20° above the horizontal. The side not to be examined is elevated 15°–20° off the table. Enough contrast material, 6–8 cc, is injected to fill the segmental bronchi of the upper lobes. Spot films are exposed. An additional 2–3 cc contrast agent is injected to outline the superior segments of the lower lobes.

After the patient is turned to the lateral decubitus position 4–5 cc contrast medium is injected to fill the lingula or the middle lobe. Spot films are exposed.

Note: The more anteriorly directed right middle lobe sometimes necessitates continued rotation of the patient toward a more prone position.

The patient is returned to the starting position (supine with the side not to be examined 15°–20° off the table) and the table is elevated toward a more erect position. An additional 5–6 cc contrast agent is injected for visualization of the segmental bronchi of the lower lobes. Spot films are exposed. The table is tilted to the horizontal position, and the overhead radiograms are exposed: AP, oblique, lateral, and delayed erect.

Note: If bilateral bronchography is performed (which should be seldom) the lateral view is omitted of the side not injected first. If a lobar or segmental bronchus is not adequately outlined during routine spot filming an additional 2–3 cc contrast material is injected in the required position so as to fill its orifice.

Selective Bronchography

Selective bronchography is utilized if a portion of the bronchial tree does not completely fill in routine bronchography, especially an atelectatic segment when bronchial neoplasm is suspected, or in recurrent segmental infiltrates.

Equipment

See "Bronchography"

Technique

The guide wire is reintroduced until it protrudes outside the catheter initially placed within the main bronchus. The catheter is removed, leaving the guide wire in position in the main bronchus. A preshaped catheter is inserted and advanced over the wire so that its tip lies at or close to the orifice of the bronchus to be entered. The wire is then removed (the catheter resumes its shape). By gentle manipulation of the catheter under fluoroscopic control the desired bronchus is selectively catheterized. Saline 2–3 cc is injected, quickly withdrawn, and placed in 50% alcohol for cytologic study.

The catheter is attached to the containing syringe, and 1–2 cc contrast agent is slowly injected at a time, until adequate visualization of the bronchial tree is obtained, injection of each bolus of contrast agent being followed by injection of a small amount of air. This precaution is necessary to insure even dispersal and coating of the walls of the bronchi by the contrast material and to avoid overfilling. However, intentional overfilling by a wedged-catheter technique has been reported to be of value in the diagnosis of emphysema.

Postprocedure Care

After removal of the catheter the soft tissues over the puncture area are gently compressed. A sterile dressing is placed over the small incision. The patient is instructed to compress the area with the finger anytime coughing occurs. Ward personnel are requested to watch for any unusual swelling of the neck or for subcutaneous emphysema. A 24-hour chest radiogram is ordered.

Contrast Laryngography

Contrast laryngography should be performed before biopsy and laryngoscopy.

Purpose

To detect benign and malignant lesions
To determine results of radiotherapy in malignant lesions
To investigate laryngomalacia, webs, cysts, laryngocele
To assess stenosis above and below the glottis
To determine status of traumatic lesions during and after therapy
To investigate functional impairment, as vocal cord paralysis
To evaluate hoarseness, mainly in patients with cancerophobia
To investigate specific areas that are inadequately seen by laryngoscopy, e.g., laryngeal ventricles, subglottic area, preepiglotic space, base of epiglottis

Contraindications

Stridor (absolute contraindication)
Very large mass lesion with insufficient airway

Filming

Cinefluoroscopy, spot films

Technique

All the various maneuvers should be explained to the patient, who should be able to perform them before the examination is begun. The patient is instructed not to cough, talk, or swallow during the examination.

Codeine 60 mg parenterally, and atropine 0.4–0.8 mg parenterally, to dry mucous membrane, are administered 1 hour before the study. An additional 0.4–0.8 mg atropine can be administered intravenously at the time of the study.

Topical anesthesia of the oropharynx and larynx is induced by spraying with 1% or 2% lidocaine (Xylocaine) while the patient breathes through the mouth. A curved metal applicator with cotton soaked in lidocaine is introduced into each piriform sinus and held there for 1 minute. An additional 2 ml of 2% lidocaine is injected by curved cannula directly over the cords and below the glottis.

Oily or aqueous propyliodone (Dionosil) or micronized barium and methylcellulose, which provide very good coating, is the contrast agent usually employed.

During quiet respiration the normal larynx is relaxed (Fig. 93a). This provides a baseline for evaluation of laryngeal anatomy and

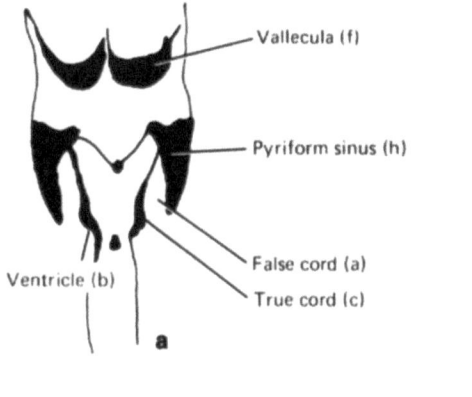

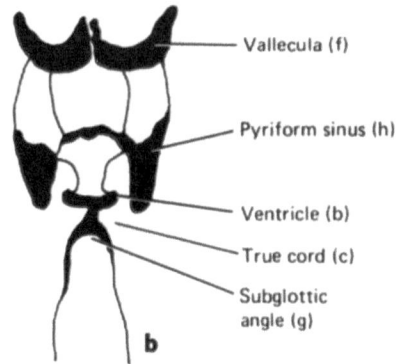

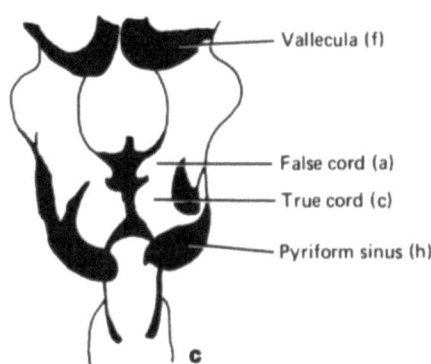

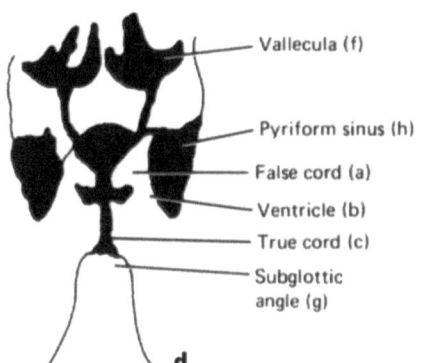

Fig. 93, a–d. Maneuvers for laryngography. **a** Larynx is relaxed during quiet respiration. **b** During phonation of EEE the AP diameter of the hypopharynx is at its maximum. **c** Phonation of AH brings vocal cords toward the midline. **d** Valsalva maneuver (forcible exhalation against the closed glottis) squares the subglottic angles.

physiology. The true and false cords are relaxed (collapsed) against the lateral walls of the larynx. The walls of the larynx are smooth and convex, and the laryngeal airway is unobstructed. The patient is then instructed to perform the various maneuvers that were previously explained.

During phonation of EEE the AP diameter of the hypopharynx is at its maximum (Fig. 93b), and full stress is placed on the vocal cords. The true cords oppose in the midline, and the false cords almost meet. The air-filled ventricles can be seen clearly, and the subglottic space is symmetrical. The piriform sinuses fill out, identifying both inner and outer laryngeal walls.

During phonation of AH partial stress is placed on the vocal cords, bringing them toward the midline of the air column (Fig. 93c).

The Valsava maneuver, which consists of forcible exhalation against the closed glottis, squares the subglottic angles (Fig. 93d).

In the modified Valsalva maneuver, air pressure causes all structures of the larynx and pharynx to balloon, resulting in excellent anatomic demonstration.

Inspiratory phonation provides the clearest depiction of the ventricles. The vocal cords are stressed downward in the reverse direction, thus yielding information about subglottic lesions.

Hysterosalpingography

Hysterosalpingography consists of roentgenography of the uterine cavity and tubal structures while they are filled with opaque material.

Purpose

To test tubal patency in infertility

To determine cause of repeated abortions, i.e., intrauterine synechia or leiomyoma, congenital uterine malformation, incompetent isthmus

To detect, after cesarean section, fistula or outpouching of the lower uterine segment

To investigate cause of abnormal uterine bleeding when dilatation and curettage showed no abnormalities, i.e., submucous leiomyoma, endometrial polyp or carcinoma, or adenomyosis

To determine if dysmenorrhea is due to uterine distension resulting from narrowing of the isthmus during follicular phase

To investigate cause of secondary amenorrhea, e.g., endometrial tuberculosis, intrauterine synechia

To localize an IUD

Contraindications

Pregnancy

Acute pelvic inflammation

Postmenopausal bleeding if carcinoma is suspected but dilatation and curettage has not been performed

Equipment

Vaginal speculum (preferably radiolucent)

No. 8 or 10 French Foley catheter (3 ml balloon)

Cervical or packing forceps

Colby adaptor

Extension tube

One 2-way stop-lock

Two 5 cc Luer Lok syringes

Water-soluble contrast material (Sinografin, Squibb)

40% Meglumine Diatrozate

20% Meglumine Iodipamdek

No. 15 needle to aspirate the contrast material from the ampule

4 × 4-in. gauze flats

Forceps and cotton sponges for preliminary cleaning

Filming

Spot films only (multiple AP and oblique spot films during injection of the contrast under fluoroscopic control)

Technique

The best time for the procedure is during the first 10 days of the menstrual cycle. It should not be performed in the premenstrual period, especially if its purpose is to study infertility (endometrial swelling may result in occlusion at the uterotubal junction). The procedure may be performed at the anticipated time of ovulation if its purpose is to study an incompetent isthmus (maximum contraction).

The patient is placed in the lithotomy position and draped as for pelvic examination. After examination of the pelvis, a speculum is inserted and the vaginal vault and cervix cleaned with thimerosal (Merthiolate) or benzalkonum (Zephiran) 1:1000.

The Foley catheter is introduced into the cervical canal with the aid of a packing forceps. It is attached to the Colby adaptor, extension tube, Luer Lok and contrast-containing syringe (10 cc). All of this is flushed through prior to attachment with the contrast medium to exclude air bubbles. The balloon on the catheter is then inflated with 1–3 cc sterile water. (Usually the balloon is inflated until mild uterine cramps signal that adequate distension has occurred or if traction on the catheter indicates that it is satisfactorily fixed within the canal. With slight traction on the catheter, contrast is injected while the progress is fluoroscopically monitored and multiple spot films are taken. The procedure can be done easily by one operator, particularly if television monitoring is used. The amount of contrast medium injected and the degree of pressure used depends upon the facility and speed of flow, and the study is terminated when all needed information is documented. Intravasation of water soluble contrast material is without significance. The speculum may be removed during the filming portion of the study.

Occasionally this technique will not succeed initially as the balloon may be extruded. Insertion higher in the isthmus will often allow completion of the study. At times, the Foley catheter technique will not succeed without a tenaculum to stabilize the cervix and allow entry of the catheter. Even more infrequently, continued extrusion of the balloon forces use of one of the older methods requiring tenaculum fixation and rigid catheters (Jarcho, Rubin, etc.) or the Swedish vacuum cannula. These methods are considerably more uncomfortable, allow less mobility in positioning the patient, usually require two operators, and cause more pain and bleeding than the Foley catheter technique.

Note: In certain cases, selective catheterization of each Fallopian tube may be accomplished under fluoroscopic control by blunt, end-hole No. 8 French catheters, introduced, if necessary, over guide wires.

Gynecography (Pelvic Pneumography)

Gynecography, roentgenography of the female reproductive tract, permits visualization of the uterine fundus ovaries, oviducts, and broad ligaments.

Purpose

To investigate polycystic ovary syndrome
To investigate Cushing's syndrome
To confirm the presence of suspected ovarian tumors and ovarian enlargement
To evaluate chronic inflammatory disease
To study endometriosis
To determine the origin of intrapelvic masses
To diagnose intersexuality early

Contraindications

Peritoneal infection
Massive hemorrhage

Equipment

Table with shoulder and boot supports (as for myelography)
Tank of nitrous oxide with attached flow meter
Two sections of latex tubing, each 2 ft long
One-way stopcock (to connect needle with the tubing)
Syringe adapter (will serve as a safety valve)
Y-shaped glass tube to connect the two sections of the tubing (The Y shape will serve as a safety valve)
No. 20 spinal needles—2 in., 3.5 in. (for obese women), and 6 in. (for patients weighing more than 300 lb)

Patient Positioning

Supine (for induction of anesthesia and introduction and removal of gas)
Prone (for filming)

Position

PA
Right anterior oblique
Left anterior oblique

Technique

The patient is given castor oil the evening before the procedure and a cleansing enema in the morning. She is not permitted anything by mouth. Seconal 100 mg is administered 1 hour before the procedure. The patient is instructed to empty her bladder before the procedure.

The patient's feet are strapped to the platform. The paraumbilical skin is prepared, and the abdomen is draped, but a small portion of the paraumbilical area is left exposed.

Local anesthesia is induced 2–4 cm to the left and below the umbilicus (in patients with left-sided scars or masses a corresponding site is chosen on the right side). A no. 20 spinal needle of proper length is used for the puncture. The needle is introduced vertically or angulated 20° toward the pelvis and slowly advanced until it enters the peritoneum. (In most instances two distinct "pops" are felt as the needle is advanced; the first may be related to puncture of the fascial planes anterior to the properitoneal fat, and the second signals entrance into the peritoneal cavity.) The obturator is removed and a 2-cc syringe attached to the needle. Aspiration is attempted to rule out inadvertent penetration of a blood vessel. If no blood is aspirated the needle is secured with a hemostat resting on the abdominal wall.

The table is tilted 25° head down. The stopcock is connected to the needle and opened to the gas line. The flow of nitrous oxide is set at 600 ml/s.

One open end of the rubber tubing is attached to the flow meter of the nitrous oxide tank. The stopcock is connected to the other open end of the tubing. The entire system is checked for leaks by occlusion of the free end of the Y-tube glass connector. The radiologist occludes the open limb of the Y-tube connector with the gloved finger and starts timing the gas flow. After a few seconds and a few times thereafter during the filling period the pressure is checked by momentarily lifting the finger from the open Y limb.

Note: Only gentle hissing should be noted. A louder noise made by the escaping gas indicates increased pressure in the system and necessitates repositioning of the needle before proceeding.

As the table is gradually tilted head down until it reaches a 45° angle, 2000–3000 ml gas is introduced over 3–5 minutes. The table is tilted down to prevent abdominal discomfort and shoulder pain, which can result from subdiaphragmatic accumulation of gas. With this precaution, the patient should experience nothing more than increasing abdominal "fullness." If the patient does complain of pain (usually as pain radiating toward the flank or epigastrium within few seconds from the onset of the gas flow), the needle is improperly placed, i.e., it is extraperitoneal, and repuncture of the peritoneal cavity is required.

Note: If there is uncertainty about the needle placement (usually in extremely stoic patients) an AP radiogram should be obtained: If the gas is intraperitoneal it sharply delineates the peritoneal cavity inferiorly and laterally. In preperitoneal injection there is a characteristic mottled appearance, and gas surrounds the bladder. If the injection is retroperitoneal there is linear dissection of the gas along the psoas shadows.

At the completion of the injection the needle is removed.

The patient is turned to the prone position and the table tilted 45° head down. With the tube at 40 in. and angled 15° toward the feet, a 14 × 17-film is exposed with the center at the anterosuperior iliac spines. (This results in a 30° pelvic inlet projection). The central beam is 3–5 cm below the tip of the sacrum.

If the radiograms are satisfactory the patient is turned to the supine position and the table tilt reduced to 25° for removal of the gas. The peritoneum is punctured through the area anesthetized earlier. A syringe containing 1 ml water or sterile saline is attached to the needle and the plunger removed. The escaping gas produces a bubbling sound. When the bubbling ceases, the needle is removed.

Postprocedure Care

The patient should remain recumbent for 2–3 hours. Occasionally a patient will complain of aching in the shoulder when sitting, but this usually disappears by the following morning. Generally follow-up observation is not necessary.

Lymphangiography

Purpose

To determine the cause of obstruction of the lymphatic circulation

To investigate cancer and other tumors of the female or male urogenital system, in particular, testicular tumors

To assess tumors of the gastrointestinal tract and of the head and neck

To investigate malignant melanomas and skin cancer

To aid in the diagnosis and management of malignant lypmhomas

Contraindications

Pulmonary disease

Right-to-left intracardiac shunt

Previous radiation therapy of lymphatics, chest, and abdomen (relative contraindication; each case be evaluated separately)

Equipment

Basic lymphangiography tray:
Lidocaine 1%
Methylene blue
Ethiodized oil (Ethiodol) 10 cc (2 ampules)
Saline solution (50 cc)
Syringes:
Two 20-cc glass
One 10-cc plastic
One 2-cc plastic
Lymphangiography needle and tubing, 30 gauge and 27 gauge (2)
Scalpel and no. 11 blade
Fine forceps with teeth
Fine forceps without teeth
Kelly clamp
Muscular clamp
Fine scissors
Small needle holder
3-0 silk
Curved cutting needles

Band-Aids
Ace bandages

Position

Vascular phase: AP, lateral, and oblique projections of both lower extremities, pelvis, and abdomen; AP view of chest
Parenchymal phase: in same projections

Technique

The patient is informed of the procedure and its complications, including the possibility of pulmonary embolus, although in the majority of cases this is asymptomatic.

The patient is brought to the radiology department on a stretcher, and everything possible should be done to make him or her comfortable since the procedure is likely to take several hours, and both feet have to be very still during the entire procedure. Valium may be administered to a restless patient.

The patient's feet are scrubbed for 10 minutes with povidone-iodine (Betadine), after which a mixture of methylene blue and lidocaine (3:1) is injected intradermally in the interdigital space with a 25-gauge needle. This may be applied in one to three spaces bilaterally. The total amount per interdigital space is 0.3 cc.

After 15 minutes a 2-cm longitudinal skin incision is made in the dorsum of each foot at the level of the first and second tarsal-metatarsal region (Fig. 94). Care should be made to avoid the prominence, which may create problems in cannulation and difficulty in healing. (Transverse skin incisions have been used by many.) A scalpel is used to incise the epidermis and dermis. Careful blunt dissection with a "mosquito" clamp permits adequate visualization of the lymphatic channels. Two 3-0 silk threads are used to isolate the lymphatic vessel. The adventitia is stripped with the fine forceps without teeth to allow dilatation and successful cannulation of the lymphatic vessel. The distal 3-0 silk is fixed to the skin under tension with a Band-Aid. Further proximal distension is accomplished by "milking" the proximal skin.

The syringe, with needle and tubing, is filled with saline or lidocaine, and the tubing is looped around the second toe to anchor the setup. The proximal lymphatic vessel is pulled up by means of the proximal 3-0 silk thread or the small pointed forceps, and the needle is inserted. At this moment saline may be injected to permit further dilatation. The lymphatic vessel is then cannulated.

The needle holder and the Band-Aid are removed, and the distal 3-0 silk thread is used to secure the needle in place. A test injection with saline is made slowly. If there is extravasation the needle is further advanced, and a knot is made with the proximal silk thread, which is then advanced cephalad to secure it. The tubing is connected to the injector and injection of Ethiodol is started. Fluoroscopy or radiography is used to follow the contrast medium in the lymphatic channels. The injection should be terminated when the upper parailiac chains are filled; in most cases 5–7 cc per side is required.

Injection of contrast agent with an automatic pressure injector takes 0.5–2 hours, according to the size of the cannulated lymphatic vessel. The same procedure can be used to assess lymphatic nodes in the axillary region.

At termination of the examination the needle and silk sutures are removed. The surgical

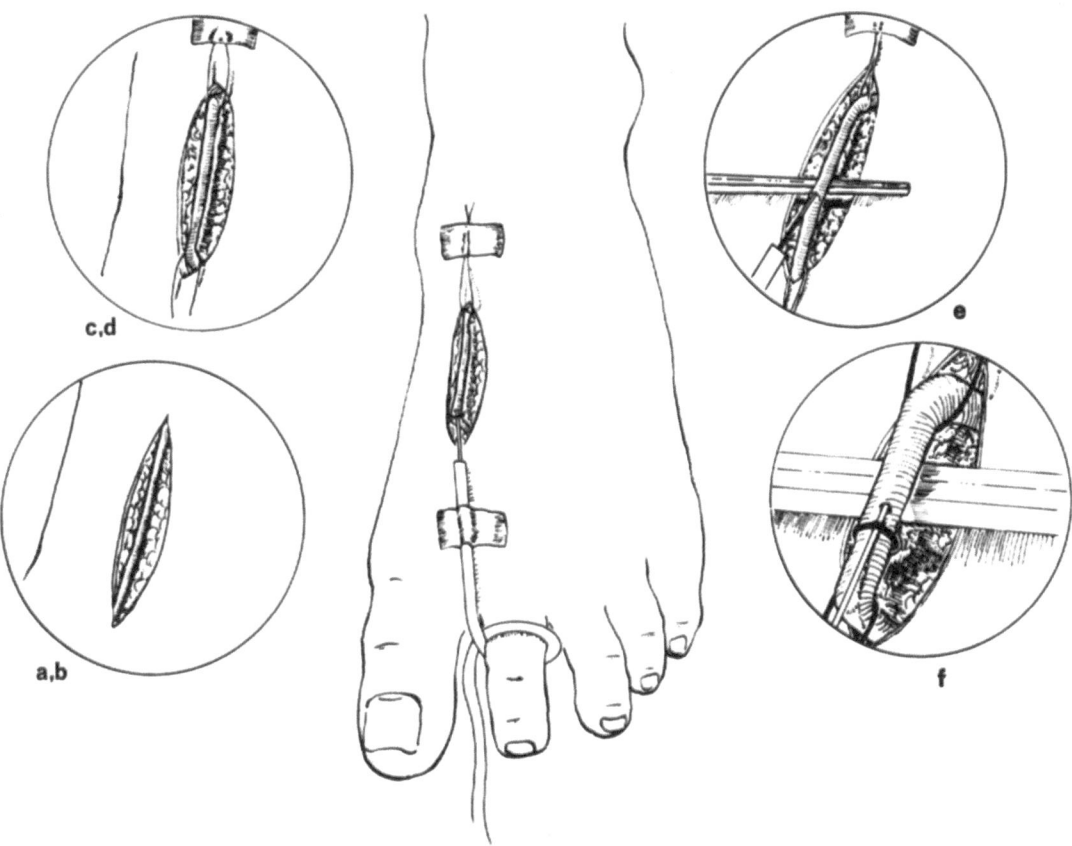

Fig. 94, a–f. Pedal lymphangiography. **a,b** Initial incision is made just below and medial to the prominence on the dorsal aspect of the foot. This incision may be made in an angle 90° to the one shown, although the vertical incision is preferred. Blunt dissection is performed to spread the incision and to isolate the lymphatic vessel. One of the most important factors in successful cannulation is to have the lymphatic vessel completely stripped of adjacent connective tissue. **c,d** Suture material is placed proximal and distal to the area of intended cannulation. The proximal suture is pulled so that some tension is exerted on the lymphatic vessel, and then the suture is taped securely. This phase may be performed by an assistant if desired. **e,f** With a forceps retracting the proximal portion of the lymphatic vessel, the vessel is cannulated, after the dorsum of the foot is massaged to help distend the lymphatic vessel (note the curling of the lymphatic catheter portion about the second toe to help secure the needle). The needle is then taped securely in place, and the proximal tie is made about the needle to secure the cannulation.

wound is thoroughly rinsed with saline solution, and the skin is sutured. A Band-Aid is used to cover the skin, and Ace bandages are applied to both feet and legs to prevent edema, which may occasionally occur after the examination.

Complications

Temporary aggravation of lymphedema
Pulmonary microemboli
Fever
Shortness of breath

7 Interventional Special Procedures

Preoperative Localization of Mammographically Demonstrated Nonpalpable Lesions of the Breasts

When the suspicious area is not palpable, localizing radiographic study minimizes the number of biopsies and decreases the amount of tissue removed for biopsy.

Purpose

To localize, for the surgeon, a breast lesion discovered by mammography as a malignant type calcification or as a mass density that is not palpable

Technique

The localizing procedure is timed, so that the biopsy will be done no later than 30 minutes after injection of the dye. The usual routine preoperative medications are administered, but local anesthesia is not used. After the original mammogram is reviewed a 22-gauge 1.5-in. needle or, if needed for depth, a 3.5-in. spinal needle is inserted into the breast (Fig. 95) at the site best estimated to place the needle tip in the center of the lesion. Craniocaudad and lateral mammograms are taken to visualize placement of the needle. If necessary the needle is adjusted to a better position within the lesion. Rarely a second set of localizing mammograms is taken if knowledge of the position is uncertain.

When the radiologist is assured of the position of the needle in the lesion, 0.5 cc of the following preparation is injected: 100 cc 1% lidocaine (Xylocaine), 100 cc normal saline, and 10 g methylene blue. This is allowed to stand for 24 hours and then autoclaved.

The surgeon removes the tissue impregnated with this dye plus a 5-mm rim. This is the lesion for frozen section. If the lesion contains calcium, specimen radiography is utilized to verify its inclusion in the specimen and to aid the pathologist in locating the best site for histoanalysis of the frozen section.

We have found this method most practical and successful, with a high degree of surgeon acceptance.

Other methods that have been suggested include:

Placement of a hooked wire at the lesion site through a needle that is then withdrawn, the hooked wire remaining in the breast while the patient is transferred to surgery

Localization of the lesion from the mammogram by extrapolation on a special diagram for the surgeon's use

Localization by skin markers

Use of two or more needles to intersect at the lesion

Use of water-soluble contrast material

Grid localization

Transhepatic Portal Venography

Purpose

To gain diagnostic information in bleeding gastroesophageal varices

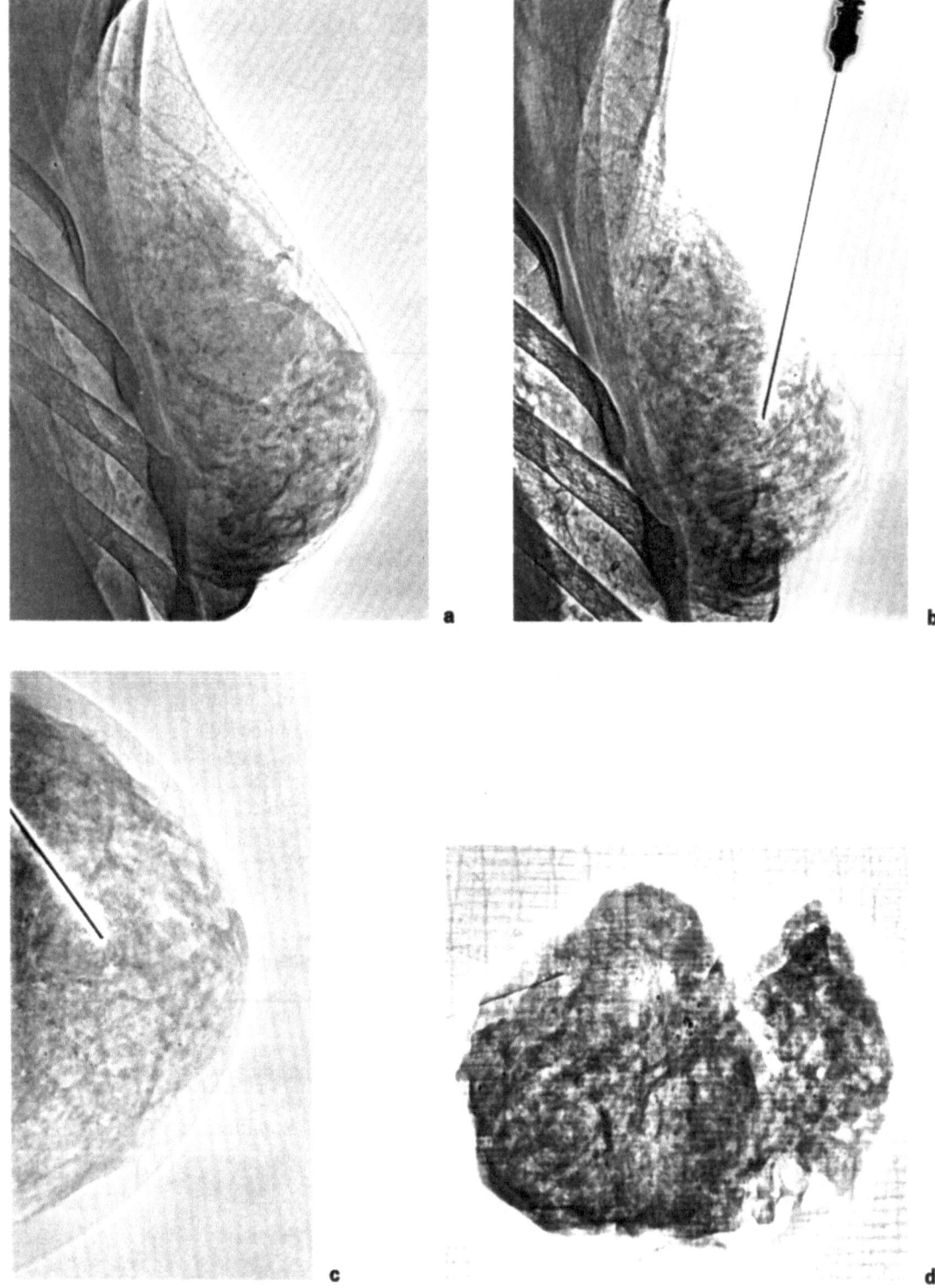

Fig. 95, a–d. Needle localization of breast lesions. Lateral xeromammogram (**a**) shows area of abnormal calcification and mass. Later (**b**) and AP (**c**) xeromammograms confirm position of tip of 20-gauge needle in the area of abnormal calcification. Specimen xeroradiograph (**d**) confirms removal of abnormal area of calcification.

To assist in therapeutic occlusion of portal vein tributaries

Injection

7–10 cc/s for 5–6 s (generally provides adequate contrast medium in the portal venous system)

Filming

Cineangiography (may be employed to provide more functional demonstration of portal venous flow)

Film Sequence

1 film/s for a total of 18 s (provides good visualization of the portal venous system and collateral vessels)

Technique

In the ideal situation an arterial portogram that localized the porta hepatis would have been done previously. Ultrasound localization of the portal vein also may be helpful.

After antiseptic preparation of the skin surface, and appropriate draping, local anesthetic is applied below the costal margin in the midaxillary line. Landmarks should be noted, and the intended needle path may be confirmed at the skin surface under fluoroscopy. After induction of local anesthesia the needle is introduced and advanced, under fluoroscopic control, toward the porta hepatis in the midaxillary line (Fig. 96). The central stylet is then removed, and gentle aspiration is attempted while the polyethylene sheath is slowly removed. When return of blood is demonstrated, a test dose of contrast medium may be injected to confirm the presence in the portal venous system. A floppy J wire is then introduced through the sheath and directed into the larger-caliber portal vein. The sheath is then advanced further into the venous system. Once placement in the portal vein is assured, appropriate measurements are obtained to provide information regarding the degree of portal hypertension (Fig. 97a). A portal venogram is then taken.

Selective catheterization of the coronary vein (Fig. 97b) and short gastric veins may be accomplished by shaping guide wires once the catheter is in the appropriate position or by use of a Cook deflector within the portal venous system.

Therapeutic Occlusion of Portal Vein Tributaries. Occlusion of the coronary vein and other sources of gastroesophageal varices has been shown to be effective in the management of variceal bleeding (Fig. 97c and d). The procedure originally described involved irritation of the venous intima with hypertonic glucose, followed by injection of thrombin, which rapidly clotted on the abnormal intima. This is readily accomplished although more difficult to control than an alternative method involving selective injection of Gelfoam emboli into the coronary vein.

Once this vein is successfully occluded the short gastric veins rapidly become more prominent and supply collateral flow to the gastroesophageal arteries. For this reason, all of the short gastric vessels must be carefully obliterated to provide a higher success rate and cessation of hemorrhage. In some patients this has resulted in spontaneous splenorenal shunts.

Transjugular Approach to the Liver (Including the Biliary System and Portal Circulation)

Select institutions have shown the transjugular approach to the liver to provide safe and effective access to the portal venous circulation as well as to the biliary tree. Furthermore, liver biopsy may be performed by this approach. (More extensive descriptions of technique and application may be found in the bibliographic entries for this section.)

Equipment

45-cm radiopaque Teflon catheter
50-cm needle with slightly curved distal portion

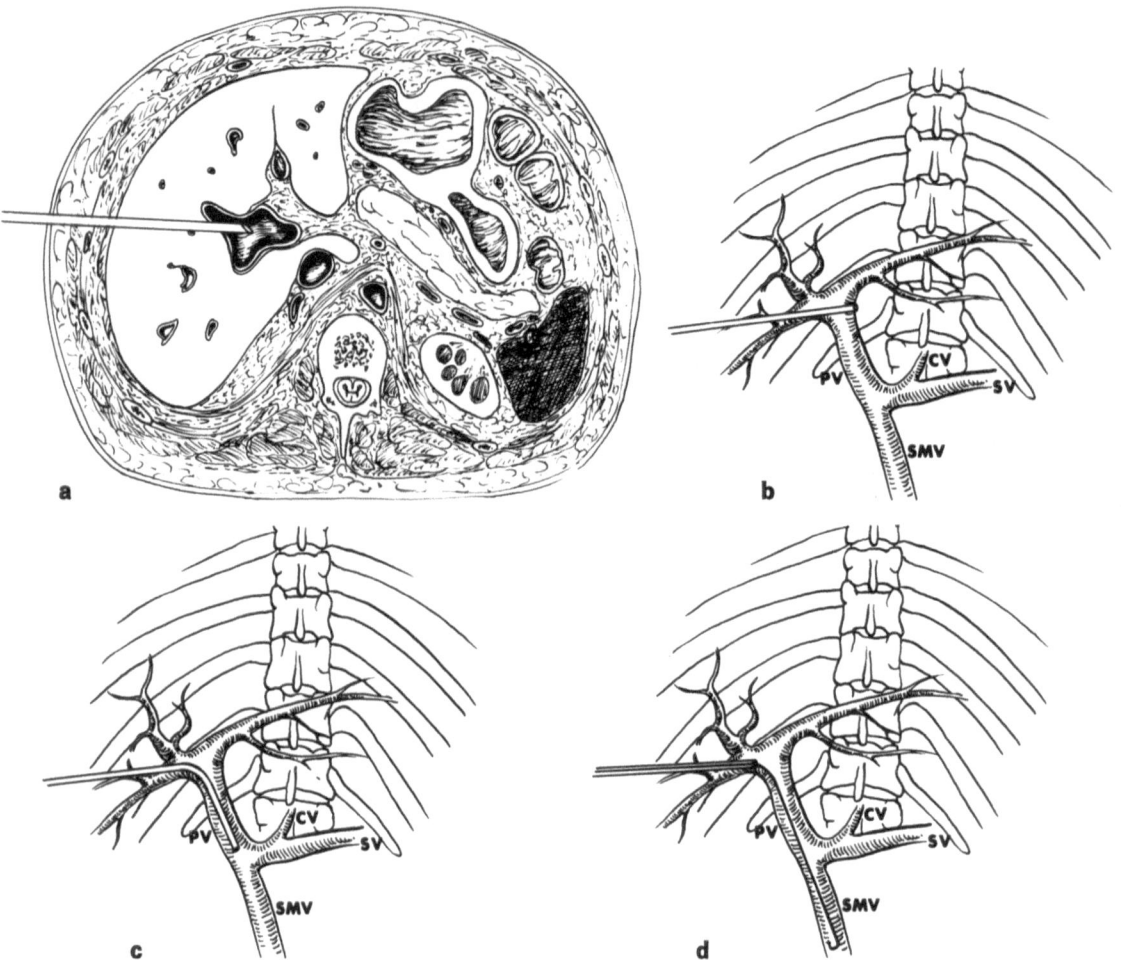

Fig. 96, a–d. Technique of transhepatic portal venography. Sheathed needle is passed into portal vein (cross section [**a**] and schematic [**b**] anterior view). After initial passage and after removal of the trocar the sheath is withdrawn. **c** The J wire is passed deep into the portal system. **d** The sheath-catheter is then removed. *PV* = portal vein; *CV* = coronary vein; *SV* = splenic vein; *SMV* = superior mesenteric vein.

Technique

A percutaneous approach is made to the internal jugular vein, preferably on the right. The puncture site is 3–4 cm below the angle of the mandible. A venous cutdown is not necessary. The catheter may be introduced into the right hepatic vein over a previously passed guide wire.

Once access is gained to the hepatic vein, numerous procedures may be performed via this approach, including hepatic venography, wedge-pressure cholangiography, liver biopsy, and portal venography.

Angiographic Diagnosis and Management of Upper Gastrointestinal Bleeding

Expeditious angiographic evaluation is extremely important in massive upper gastrointestinal bleeding, because of the critical state of the patient. Every evaluation should be complete, even though the source of the bleeding is believed to be known, e.g., duodenal ulcer or esophageal varices. A complete examination includes demonstration of the left gastric and gastroduodenal arteries, preferably by subselective injection. In addition, the superior mesenteric artery is visualized with an enhanced portal venous phase demonstrated. Since bleeding may be from other sites in more than 30% of patients with known esophageal varices, arterial hemorrhage must be ruled out before splenic vasospasm is initiated for treatment of the gastroesophageal varices.

Demonstration of extravasation of contrast medium from the arterial system into the gastrointestinal lumen or other spaces is diagnostic of arterial hemorrhage. In the absence of gross extravasation, marked mucosal blush and prominent venous filling may occasionally demonstrate hemorrhagic gastritis.

Technique

When arterial hemorrhage is demonstrated angiographically the catheter should be placed as close to the bleeding vessel as possible (left gastric, gastroduodenal). When duodenal bleeding is demonstrated, subselective catheterization of the gastroduodenal artery is ideal. In some cases, however, this may not be possible, and perfusion of the celiac axis or common hepatic artery may be an alternative. This represents some risk, especially in cirrhotic patients with hepatic ischemia. Superior mesenteric arterial infusion, with the catheter tip close to or in the origin of the inferior pancreaticoduodenal artery, is therefore suggested. Since the duodenum is supplied by a dual vascular bed, infusion from either side has been effecitve. Evaluation of collateral flow at the time of diagnostic angiography may provide prognostic information regarding the success of this maneuver, that is, if a dual blood supply is demonstrated angiographically, perfusion of the superior mesenteric artery will generally result in vascular constriction of the duodenum.

An infusion of vasopressin (Pitressin) 0.1–0.2 U/minute is then initiated and continued for 20 minutes. A control angiogram is obtained following this trial. If vasospasm and cessation of hemorrhage are incomplete, extravasation of contrast medium persists, and transcatheter therapeutic embolization may then be considered (see next section).

It is important that flow rates and timing of the film sequence be consistent in both of these infusions.

Gastroesophageal varices. In patients with portal hypertension, blood flow is increased in the portal venous system and distribution of the coronary vein. Perfusion of the superior mesenteric artery will result in a secondary reduction in venous flow. Catheterization should not be superselective because this increases the risk of intestinal ischemia. A control angiogram should be obtained after 20 minutes to confirm the presence of vasospasm. It has been demonstrated that Pitressin may actually increase hepatic blood flow. Therefore when reversal of flow (visualization of the portal vein) is demonstrated on the hepatic arteriogram, serious consideration should be given to the fact that perfusion of the superior mesenteric artery may actually increase the flow to the esophageal varices because of the increased flow through the liver.

Vasopressin infusion in gastrointestinal hemorrhage

Vasopressin mix

$$\frac{100 \text{ U vasopressin (Pitressin-S)}}{500 \text{ cc normal saline}} = 0.2 \text{ U/cc}$$

$$1 \text{ cc} = 15 \text{ drops} = 60 \text{ microdrops}$$

Arterial hemorrhage

1) Demonstration of active extravasation of contrast
2) Selective vasopressin infusion (0.1–0.2 U) for 20 minutes
3) Repeat angiography with the same injection and filming factors

If hemorrhage has stopped, infusion is continued for 6–12 hours, then infusion rate is gradually reduced. Infusion of normal saline is generally continued for 12 hours after cessation of hemorrhage in case of rebleeding.

If hemorrhage continues, dose is increased to a maximum of 0.4 U/minute. If hemorrhage has not stopped or is not markedly reduced, therapeutic embolization or surgery* should be considered.

---

* Relative contraindication to selective hepatic infusion.

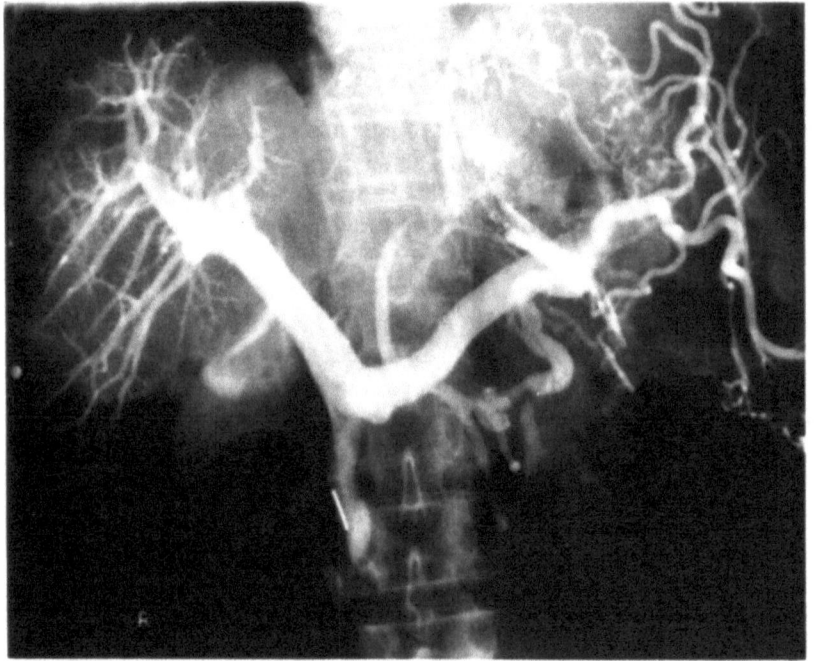

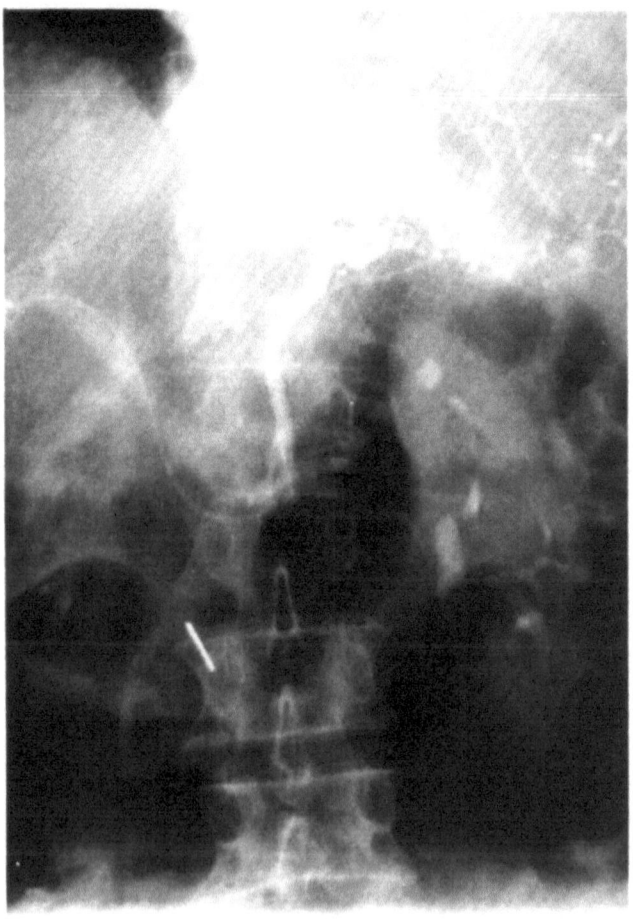

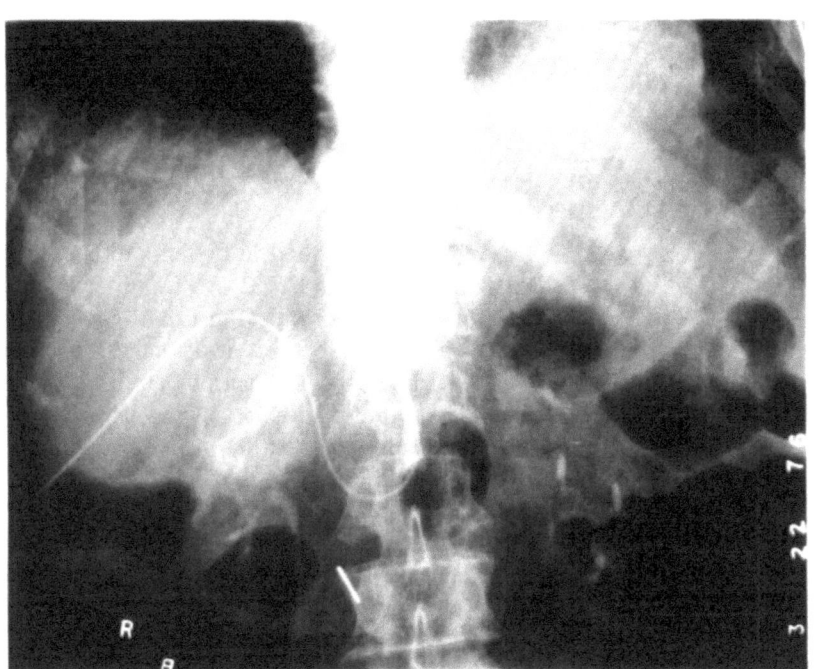

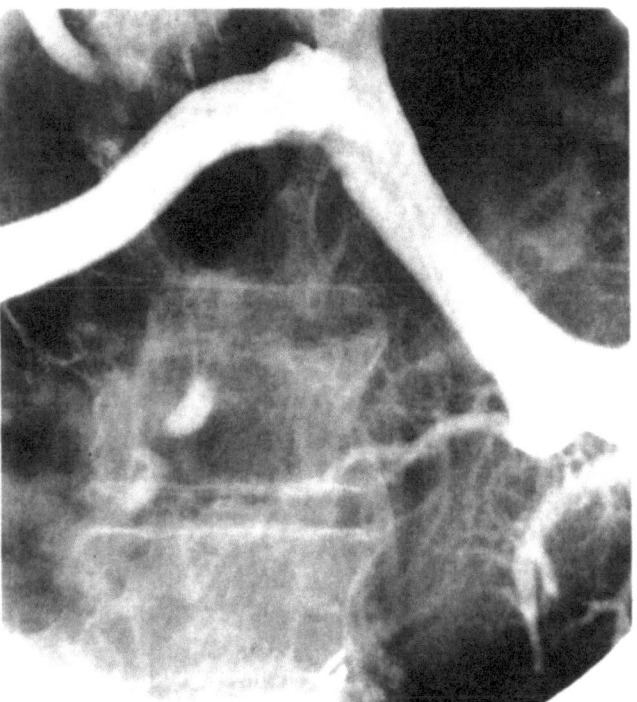

Fig. 97, a–d. Transhepatic portal venography and obliteration of esophageal varices. **a** Transhepatic portal venogram showing portal venous anatomy with portal pressure of 400 mm H$_2$O. **b** Selective catheterization of the coronary vein shows more clearly the marked gastroesophageal varices. **c** Following Gelfoam embolization, obliteration of the varices is demonstrated with residual patency of the body of the coronary vein. **d** Portal venogram following additional embolization demonstrates complete obliteration of the coronary vein.

4)   If hemorrhage is from the duodenum, the pancreatic or duodenal arcade should be evaluated. Often infusion of the superior mesenteric access near the inferior pancreatic or duodenal artery will provide the same physiologic result as selective gastroduodenal artery infusion.

Transcatheter Therapeutic Embolization

Massive hemorrhage from the gastrointestinal tract and other sites is often demonstrated angiographically. Infusion of vasopressor substances has been extremely helpful in controlling hemorrhage from the gastrointestinal tract, but there have been failures due to various factors. In addition, bleeding may be from vessels in which catheter position is tenuous or from vessels that respond poorly to vasopressors.

Purpose

To provide a definitive mode of cessation of hemorrhage

Numerous methods of arterial occlusion have been devised, including injection of autologous clots, with or without additives; Silastic pellets; muscle fragments; silicone rubber; and Gelfoam. In addition, mechanical methods of occlusion, including use of balloon catheters and cotton threads, have been described. All of these methods have inherent advantages and disadvantages.

In general, I prefer to use Gelfoam in the treatment of arterial hemorrhage because the size of the embolus can be readily controlled and because Gelform can be used in various sized catheters. Disadvantages are that occlusion of large-caliber vessels is somewhat difficult with small Gelfoam plugs and Gelfoam emboli last longer than autologous clots. In one patient, autologous fat emboli were employed, and in another, autologous clots. Also used are small fragments of Gelfoam, injected several at a time. This method is useful for occlusion of small vessels and in arteriovenous malformations.

Equipment

Gelfoam strips 2×5 mm
Small syringe 2.5–10 cc
Scalpel blade

Technique

Gelfoam is supplied in a standard sterilized pad of 2×6 cm; dry 2- $\times$ 5-mm strips are cut on the sterile tray (Fig. 98). The size is extremely variable, and it is suggested that trials be made through various sized catheters used in the angiographic suite. The strips become difficult to work with once they are moist, so moistness should be avoided.

A single plug is placed at the nozzle of a small syringe with the plunger removed. Contrast material is poured into the syringe and the plunger replaced. The syringe is connected to the catheter adapter and the embolus injected. The Gelfoam plug has a lower specific gravity than the contrast agent and will float to the surface; therefore inversion of the syringe will allow easy passage into the catheter. Once the plug is in place, continuous pressure must be applied to eject the embolus from the catheter.

Percutaneous Lung Biopsy

Percutaneous lung biopsy is a relatively safe nonsurgical procedure. Not only can lung tissue be obtained for microscopic evaluation, but bacteriologic and other laboratory examinations may be performed on the aspirate. Fluoroscopic guidance of the needle will assure its precise placement at the site of the lung lesion.

Purpose

To assess a mass lesion 1.0 cm or more
To evaluate lung patterns
To study infiltrates of questionable cause

Technique

Aspiration biopsy of a lung lesion relies heavily on high-quality cytologic evaluation, and cooperation with the pathology department is extremely important in increasing the accuracy of diagnosis. Immediate preparation of the specimen is necessary to ensure good quality diagnostic material.

A 19–23-gauge needle may be used successfully. The lesion should be approached from the skin surface closest to it, which thus reduces the needle path through normal lung. The lesion is located by fluoroscopy, and the skin over it is marked. Biplane fluoroscopy and C-arm fluoroscopy, which moves into both planes, are ideal. If these are not available, however, depth of the lesion may be approximated before aspiration from a lateral radiograph and confirmed by a lateral projection during the procedure.

Local anesthetic administered at the site of anticipated needle placement results in formation of a superficial wheal. Infiltration to the pleural surface is made at the puncture site. It is preferable for the needle to course over the superior aspect of a rib rather than the inferior aspect where the intercostal vessels are located. After passage through subcutaneous tissue the needle with a holder is advanced, under fluoroscopic control, during suspended respiration. If the radiologist prefers holding the needle with the fingers, intermittent fluoroscopy may be used.

After the needle is at the appropriate depth, an exposure is made at a plane 90° to the needle path to confirm the position of the tip within the suspected lesion. Once this is confirmed the patient is instructed not to breathe, and the stylet is quickly withdrawn and a finger applied to the needle opening. A high-suction syringe is then attached, and suction is applied. The plunger may be withdrawn and advanced to provide intermittent suction, following which the entire apparatus is withdrawn. The needle (without the stylet) may be moved up and down a few millimeters to help disrupt some of the abnormal tissue and ease aspiration of tissue.

If pneumothorax is not present this process may be repeated up to three times, and it may be repeated at another session if diagnostic information is not obtained.

Since this material is sufficient only for cytological or microbiological evaluation, the slides are generally prepared at the time of aspiration, being smeared and sprayed with

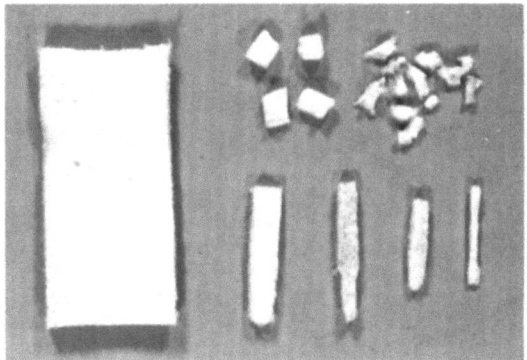

Fig. 98.   Cut Gelfoam strips on sterile tray.

100% alcohol. In the ideal situation the cytologist is present at the biopsy.

Screw Needle Apparatus for Obtaining Material for Cytologic Study

Introduced by Nordenstrom, a stainless-steel screw needle 0.55 mm in diameter that fits through a stainless-steel cannula 1 mm in diameter (Ursus Konsult AB, Barrtorpsvagen 9, S-150 24 Ronninge, Sweden) (Fig. 99). It may be used in lung lesions as well as for sampling from liver, kidney, lymph nodes, and mammary tumors. The needle is quite fine and obtains material of better quality for cytologic study than is obtained by simple aspiration.

Technique

Under fluoroscopic control the cannula needle apparatus (with screw portion in position) is placed to the edge of the suspicious lesion. The outer cannula and instrument holder are held in place while the screw needle is rotated clockwise until it is completely inserted. With the screw fixed in the same position, the cannula is rotated counterclockwise while being advanced over the screw portion. At the completion of this maneuver the cannula should be completely over the screw portion. The entire apparatus is then removed, and the screw needle is pushed out of the tip of the cannula. The needle should not be pulled out of the

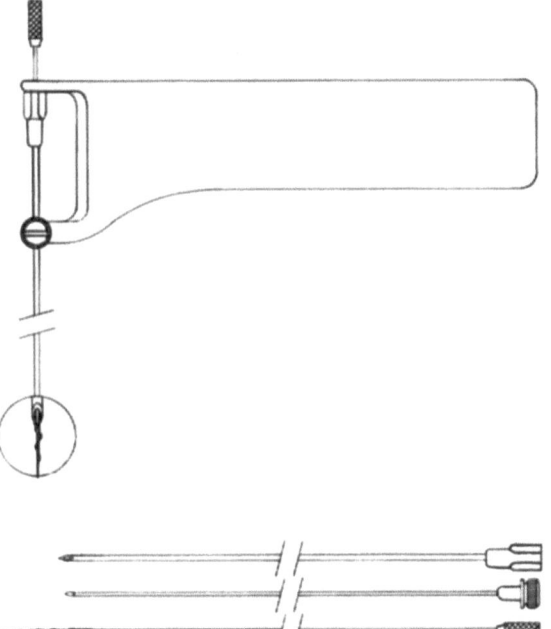

Fig. 99. Screw needle apparatus. Surgimed, Inc., U.S.A.

cannula because cell material will be lost within the cannula.

Advantages of this technique, as pointed out by Nordenstrom, are:

1) Material is obtained over a greater distance, i.e., 15 mm, the length of the screw portion.
2) Some fixation in the lesion is produced by the screw, and organized abnormalities, especially granuloma, may be adequately sampled.
3) Additional material, such as connective tissue, may be sampled, which may be of diagnostic value.

Cutting-Needle Biopsy

Because cutting needles are of significantly larger caliber than other needles and actually cut tissue, the risk of pneumothorax is greater with their use. The amount of tissue obtained, however, is significantly larger, and thus the risk of procuring insufficient tissue for diagnosis is reduced.

Numerous needles may be used for cutting biopsy, including the Vim-Silverman cutting needle and a needle used for prostatic biopsy. These are particularly adaptable to large lesions in the pleural where the risk of pneumothorax is less because of the anatomic site.

Patients may expectorate blood or blood-tinged sputum for a short period after biopsy. This is good material for cytologic study and should be sent to the laboratory for the 24 hours following biopsy. PA and lateral chest roentgenograms are usually obtained immediately after, 2–3 hours after, and 24 hours after biopsy. Although certain factors and pulmonary findings after biopsy may alter this.

Nonoperative Extraction of Retained Biliary Calculi

Three procedures, which utilize a basket, a catheter, or both, are currently available for extraction of biliary calculi retained after cholecystectomy, thereby saving the patient a second operation with its significantly higher morbidity and mortality. All may be done on an ambulatory basis, however hospitalization is preferred to allow a course of intravenous antibiotics during the manipulation.

Extraction of biliary calculi is technically easy to master, being easiest in relatively thin patients in which the drainage tract is short and straight and the T tube large (14–16 F). The latter is an important point to emphasize to surgeons. In order to have a good fibrous tract through which to carry out the necessary manipulations it is essential to wait 4–6 weeks postoperatively before the procedure is attempted. This period also gives smaller stones an opportunity to pass spontaneously.

Moderate sized calculi are the easiest to extract—small stones (less than 2–3 mm), which can pass spontaneously, and large stones (greater than 1.2–1.5 cm) are more difficult to "capture." The very large stones are difficult to pull through the sinus tract. However, the basket can be used to break up the larger stones into sizes that are more manageable.

Purpose

To remove retained biliary (intrahepatic or common-duct) calculi confirmed by postoperative T-tube cholangiography

Contraindications

No absolute contraindications
Local skin or wound infection (minor relative
    contraindication)

Equipment

Dormia (ureteral) baskets (9 and 15 mm) with
    Teflon sheaths
A steerable polyethylene catheter system, cath-
    eter sizes 8.5 and 13 F (Burhenne Biliary
    Stone Removal System, Meditech, Water-
    town, Massachusetts) (The system permits
    injection of contrast agent and basket ma-
    nipulation.)
Standard angiographic catheters (10–12 F)
    with a short simple curve at the tip (These
    catheters are a reasonable alternative to the
    steerable catheter system.)
Angiographic guide wires (both straight and
    J shaped) with movable cores (These may
    be necessary if angiographic catheters are
    to be used instead of the steerable system.)

Technique (Figs. 100 and 101)

At the end of the 4–6 week period after
cholecystectomy T-tube cholangiography is performed to confirm the number and location of
stones. Premedication is not necessary, but in
a very anxious patient 5 mg diazepam (Valium) can be administered intravenously. If the
tract is very tortuous or the stone impacted distally, intramuscular administration of 50 mg
meperidine (Demerol) may occasionally be
necessary to relieve pain during manipulations
and instrumentation.

A broad-spectrum antibiotic such as am-
picillin (1 gm orally four times a day) should
be administered on the day prior to the procedure and for 2–3 days afterward, if performed on an outpatient.

Administration of glucagon 1–2 mg intravenously may induce hypotonicity and sphincter relation. This is especially helpful if pushing small to moderate-sized stones through the
papilla is being considered.

Diatrizoate meglumine and diatrizoate sodium (Renografin-60) or diatrizoate (Hypaque 50% diluted with an equal volume of
normal saline is the contrast agent used.

If the Burhenne system is to be used the
T tube can be removed and the skin prepared.
A sterile field should be maintained. The steerable catheter is maneuvered into the common
duct distal to the stone(s). If the stone is in an
intrahepatic radicle, it should be manipulated
into the common duct where it is easier to
handle. This is done with the catheter or by
positioning of the patient.

The Dormia basket together with its Teflon
sheaths is inserted into the steerable catheter
up to its distal tip. Advancing the basket beyond the steerable catheter can result in ductal

Fig. 100, a–f. Retrieval of
stone retained in the common
bile duct (after Burhenne).
a Calculus is demonstrated
after T tube has been left in
place for 4–6 weeks. **b** T tube
is removed. **c** Catheter is
placed through the fistula and
guided into the common bile
duct. **d** Retrieval basket is
inserted through the catheter.
e After manipulation of the
apparatus in the common bile
duct the stone is within the
basket. **f** Basket-stone-catheter
apparatus is removed (the
stone will often be frag-
mented, especially if the
fistula tract is small).

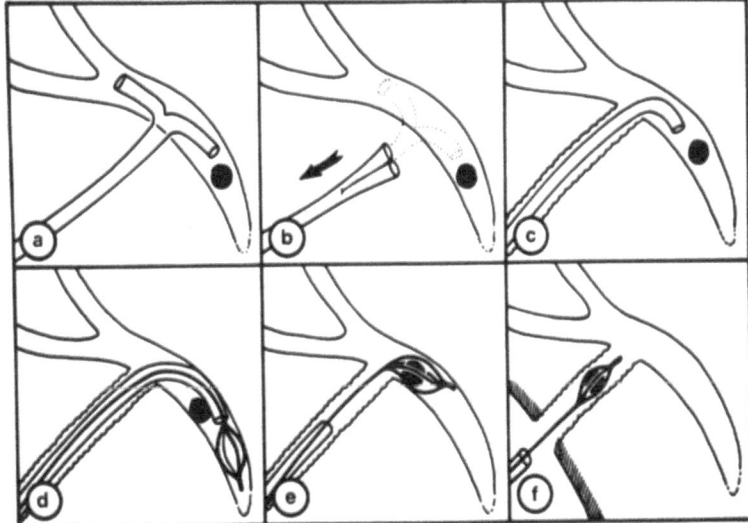

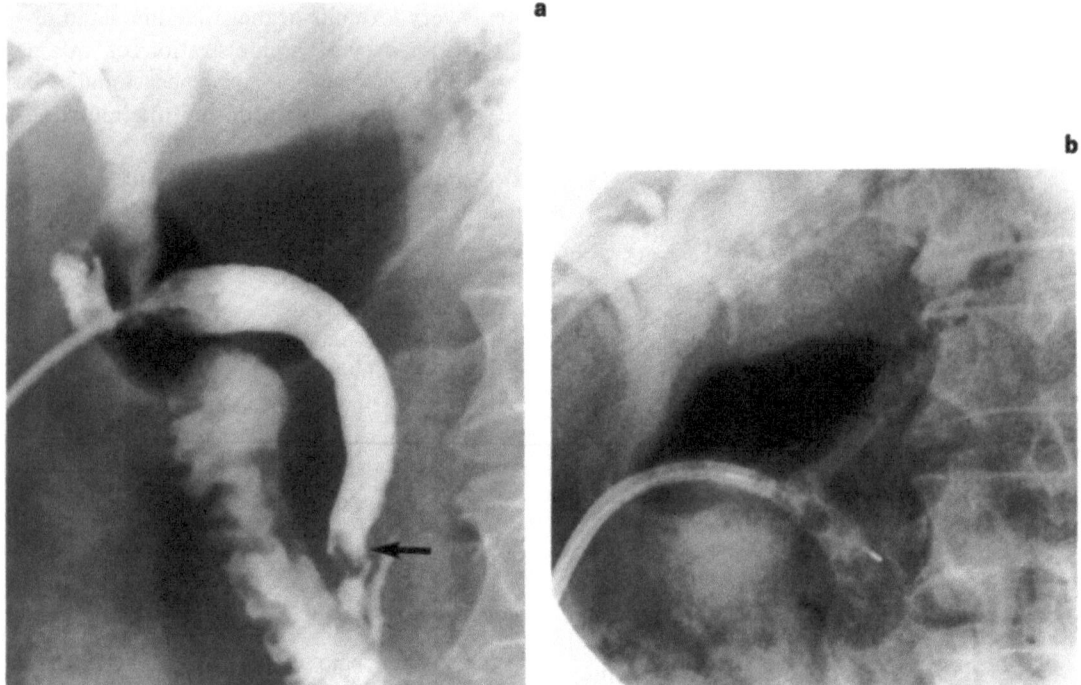

Fig. 101, a and **b.**   Retrieval of stone retained in the common bile duct. **a** Injection of contrast material within the tube demonstrates a 1-cm calculus (*arrow*) in the distal common blie duct. **b** Calculus (*arrow*) lies within the basket of the catheter-basket apparatus.

injury, including perforation. The steerable catheter and then the Teflon sheath are withdrawn approximately 3–4 cm to permit the basket to open. The basket is pulled back to capture the stone (rotation of the basket may be necessary). The basket containing the stone is pulled snug against the Teflon sheath, and the entire system, including the steerable catheter, is withdrawn.

This procedure can be repeated many times if multiple stones are present.

If the Burhenne system is not used a large angiographic catheter (10 F) can be used. This may be useful in patients with small tortuous tracts. However, the catheter may be difficult to reinsert after the initial attempt at extraction. The T tube is not removed at the beginning of the procedure.

The skin and T tube are prepared. A J-shaped guide wire is inserted into the common duct via the T tube, after which the T tube is removed. The angiographic catheter is passed over the guide wire, which is then removed. The wire basket with its Teflon sheath is in-

serted, and the stone is captured and removed in the same manner as with the Burhenne system.

Another method for removing small, distal biliary calculi consists of insertion of a straight rubber catheter (10–12 F) into the common duct, administration of glucagon, and pushing the stones through into the duodenum after sphincter relaxation.

Regardless of which procedure is used, at its termination it is necessary to insert a straight rubber (14–16 F) catheter into the common duct to provide drainage, particularly in difficult extractions in which there may be significant papillary edema, and to provide a means for a final postprocedure study of the biliary tree.

Complications

Mild pain during instrumentation and injection of contrast medium (similar to that in T-tube studies) and if large stones have to be extracted through the sinus tract

Occasionally a low-grade temperature immediately after the procedure (This can be largely eliminated with the use of broad-spectrum antibiotics.)

Rarely perforation of the common duct or the fibrous sinus tract

Retrieval of Intravascular Foreign Bodies

With the increasing use of intravascular catheters ("intracaths") and central venous pressure monitoring by the general house staff in both intensive care units and general medical and surgical services, there have been increasing reports of dislodgment of portions of the polyethelene catheters. The fragments may then be contained within the peripheral venous system or may circulate toward the heart and be deposited in the cardiac chambers or pulmonary circulation. Occasionally guide wires used in angiography may break as a result of faulty technique and cause similar problems.

In almost all instances of intravascular foreign bodies, a technical error was made in placement of the intracath—either in the initial placement or in attempts to change the position of the central venous pressure (CVP) catheter line. Most important in this regard is never to pull back on the intracath through the overlying needle, which has a very sharp cutting edge, and subsequently sever the catheter portion. For this reason and because the inci-

dence of phlebitis associated with the use of intracaths is significantly high, CVP catheters should be placed only when they are clearly indicated. Furthermore, they should not be manipulated once they are in place, and central venous pressure lines should be frequently changed to avoid phlebitis and systemic infection.

Retained intravascular foreign bodies may be asymptomatic, but complications have been reported, among them venous obstruction and secondary thromboembolic phenomena, including pulmonary emboli. Portions of the catheter may lodge in the myocardium and cause its rupture, be a nidus for bacterial infection, or occasionally result in valvular dysfunction. The ideal time to attempt removal of a foreign body is as soon as dislodgement has occurred.

Among the devices reported to remove intravascular foreign bodies are snares or loops, hook catheters, and forceps of various types. One of two situations generally determines the method of foreign body removal: a catheter can be manipulated (1) to the tip (either end) of the foreign body or (2) to the central portion of the foreign body.

Snare or Loop Retrieval

Equipment

8 F catheter with end-hole only
0.025 double-length guide wire with central portions floppy (Fig. 102)

Fig. 102, a–d. Snare method of foreign body retrieval.
a Intravascular foreign body lies within the right atrium.
b Snare apparatus consists of a long guide wire that forms a loop when passed through an 8 F catheter. **c** A considerable amount of wire is placed around the foreign body. (This degree of looping is generally not necessary.) **d** The wire is then withdrawn until the foreign body is snared at the catheter tip.

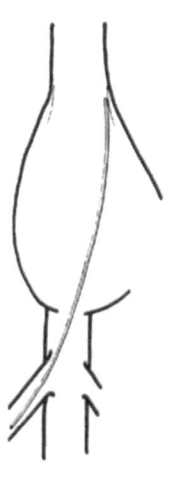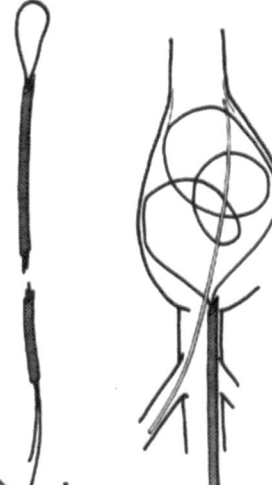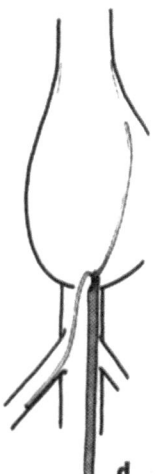

Technique

The wire is folded and inserted through the catheter with both ends of the wire remaining outside of the catheter. Movement of the ends of the wire separately or together changes the size and direction of the loop. After the catheter assembly is manipulated to the foreign body, the loop is opened and the foreign body snared. After the loop is closed around the foreign body the entire assembly is removed transfemorally.

Use of a sheath (Desilets) will facilitate removal of the entire assembly and reduce trauma to the vein on extraction.

Hook Catheter Retrieval

When access cannot be gained to the end of the foreign body, a deflector-catheter assembly may be used to "hook" the foreign body (Fig. 103). If the foreign body is not entirely removed by this method the snare technique may have to be used in conjunction with it.

Both of these techniques may be modified by individual ingenuity.

Transluminal Angioplasty

Although described in 1963, it is only recently that percutaneous transluminal angioplasty has gained some acceptance, largely due to considerable experience in Europe and development of a balloon catheter for dilatation (Grüntzig). Angioplasty is now an accepted mode of therapy for peripheral vascular disease of specific types and will make a great impact on the nonoperative treatment of renovascular hypertension. In addition, promise has been shown in the treatment of atherosclerotic coronary vascular disease.

In performing percutaneous transluminal angioplasty, one accepts a greater role in patient management and the incumbent responsibilities of a therapist, in addition to those of a diagnostician.

Dotter Technique

Femoral Artery Dilatation. Transluminal dilatation of stenosed arteries of the lower extremity, most commonly the superficial femoral artery, employs a coaxial system of catheters (Fig. 104) and involves progressive dilatation of the arterial lumen, without extravasation, plowing, or reaming.

Purpose

To dilate short stenosed segments of the superficial femoral artery

To recanalize arterial lumen (short segments)

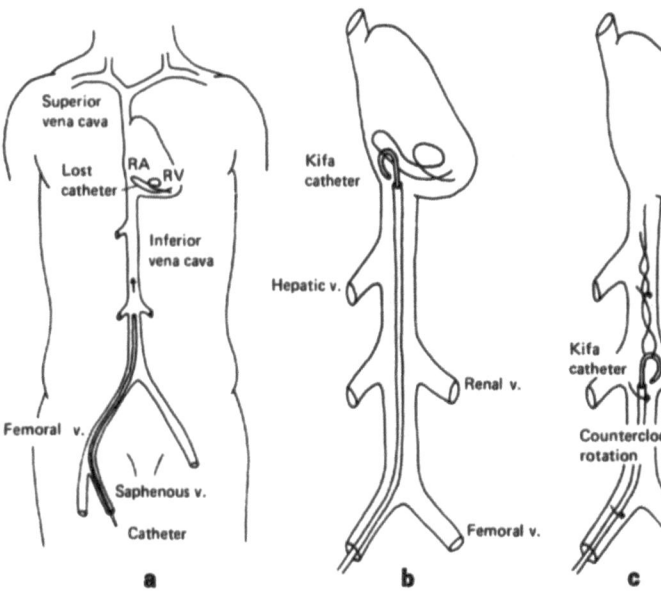

Fig. 103, a–c. Hook method of foreign body retrieval. **a** A catheter is placed percutaneously into the inferior vena cava to retrieve a coiled foreign body within the right atrium (*RA*) and right ventricle (*RV*). b A second hook catheter or deflector wire is used to hook the foreign body. **c** After retrieval of the foreign body it is brought into the inferior vena cava.

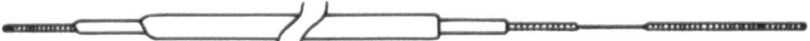

Fig. 104. The Dotter transluminal dilatation set. Courtesy of Cook Incorporated

when there is complete occlusion in patients with gangrene.

To dilate stenotic segments of deep femoral artery

Equipment

5 F polyethylene diagnostic catheter
0.038 wire
0.045 guide wire
8 F and 12 F dilating catheters

Technique

In our experience the most difficulty initially is in making the optimal anterograde puncture because the landmarks for retrograde puncture of the common femoral artery are generally more familiar. Since the needle will be directed toward the lower extremity the incision and original skin entry site must be considerably higher than the site conventionally used for femoral artery puncture. Fluoroscopic localization of landmarks may be compared with previous angiograms to pinpoint the site of puncture. If the site is too distal the deep femoral artery or the superficial femoral artery itself will be punctured, and if the latter is discased at its orifice, further advancement of the wire may be difficult.

Once the puncture is made a straight conventional guide wire and subsequently a 5 F straight catheter are passed into the superficial femoral artery. Control angiograms are obtained and the distal runoff evaluated. These are important for comparison after angioplasty.

After angiography the 6 F diagnostic catheter is replaced with a rigid Teflon 8 F dilating catheter. A .045 guide wire and subsequently an 8 F dilating catheter are passed through the stenotic area. The catheter is then withdrawn to a level above the stenosis, and fluoroscopic evaluation is repeated.

In severe stenosis, this procedure will undoubtedly produce considerable improvement, but the lumen will be dilated only to 8 F. A stiff 12 F dilating catheter is then placed over the 8 F catheter and introduced to the arterial lumen. The wire is passed through the stenotic area, followed by the 8 F and then the 12 F catheter. The 12 F catheter may be rotated somewhat at this time. Resistance to the catheter usually signals passage through the stenotic area. The entire system is then brought more proximally, and control angiograms are again obtained. Time is a factor in success of the procedure, especially when the superficial femoral artery is small and the 12 F catheter itself may be causing some occlusion. Prior to withdrawal of the apparatus, 3000 U heparin may be instilled proximal to the dilated segment.

Before the catheter is removed dilatation of the diseased segment and distal runoff are documented by angiography. We also make biplane studies of the diseased segment before and after dilatation for complete documentation. After completion of the procedure and documentation the apparatus is removed, and the site of the arterial puncture is closed by manual compression.

Iliac Artery Dilatation.   Transluminal dilatation has been extremely successful in mild to severe iliac artery stenoses. Many consider it the procedure of choice in iliac artery stenosis because of its relative ease and speed and the lengthy recovery time associated with surgery.

Purpose

To dilate stenosed segment of the iliac artery (without occlusion)

Equipment (Fig. 105)

6 F polyethylene straight catheter
.038 floppy straight guide wire
8 F cage catheter
Inflatable balloon catheter
8 F diagnostic catheter

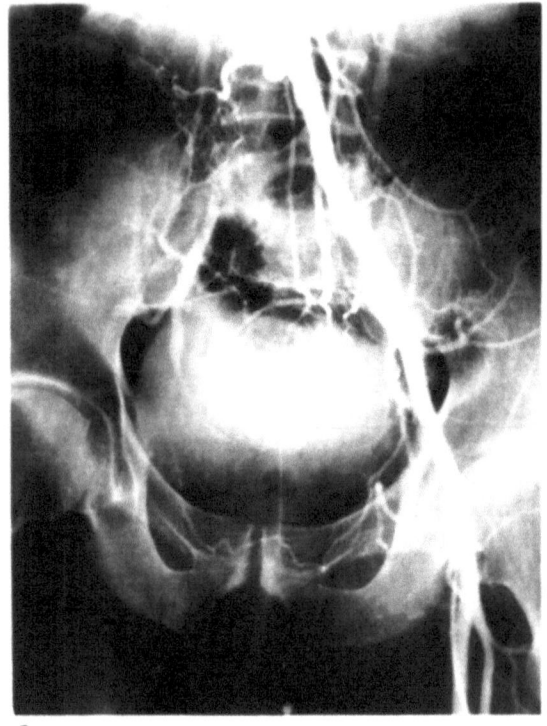

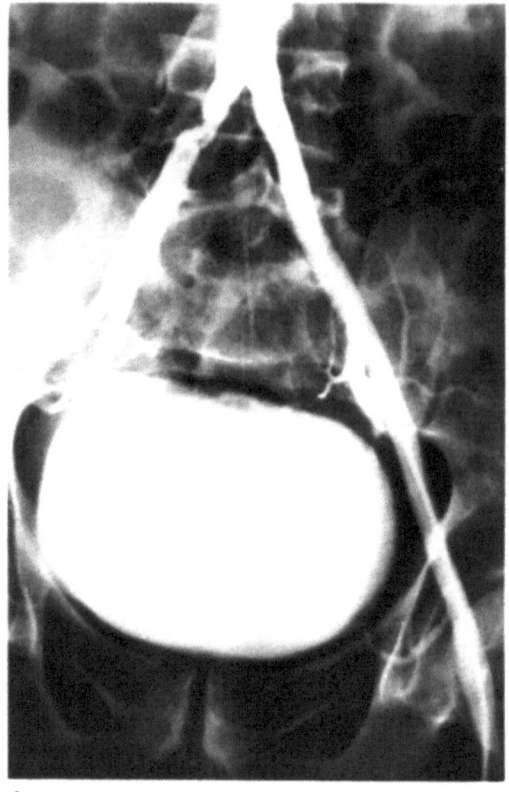

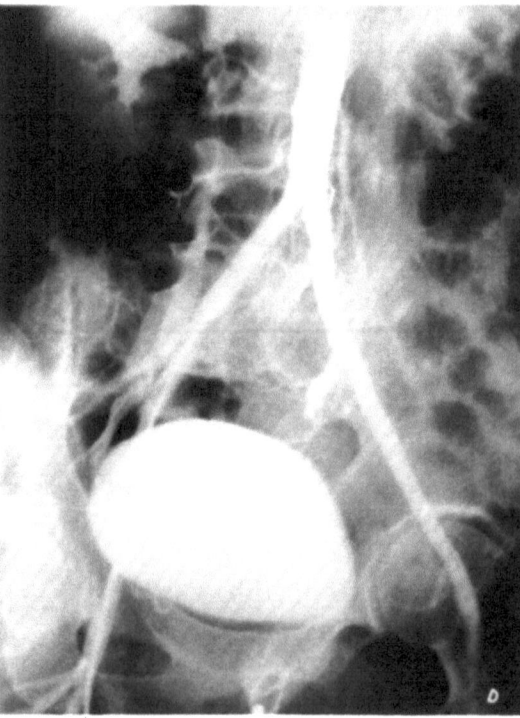

Fig. 105, a–c. Transluminal dilatation of the iliac artery. **a** Injection of contrast material at the bifurcation of the aorta demonstrates complete occlusion of the right common iliac artery. **b** After 23 hours of streptokinase infusion (5000 U/hour) a short stenotic lesion is demonstrated. **c** After balloon dilatation of the artery the arteriogram shows the lumen to be almost normal.

Technique

In confirmed iliac artery stenosis the common femoral artery on the ipsilateral side of the stenosis is punctured in the conventional manner after induction of local anesthesia. A standard guide wire is introduced and gently advanced toward the lower abdominal aorta, traversing the stenotic area. A conventional straight diagnostic aortography catheter (5–6 F) is placed in the lower abdominal aorta in the usual manner.

At this time, even if arteriography was performed recently, a control angiogram is obtained. Dotter used the contralateral femoral artery and an additional catheter for this control angiogram; howeyer, this is at the discretion of the operator. Pressures may be obtained on both sides of the stenosis to document the severity of gradient. During the initial wire and catheter placement, extreme care must be taken not to use force and pass the wire subintimally.

Heparin sodium 3000 U is employed for low-dose systemic heparinization. Since advancement through the groin will cause buckling of the catheter cage, a thin polyester sheath is used to pass the 8 F cage catheter. This will provide support and keep the cage closed during the insertion.

As described by Dotter, the dilatation may be performed in one of two ways:

1) For stenoses more than 1 cm long. The conventional guide wire is replaced by the balloon cannula, which is manufactured so that the balloon will be placed exactly in the caged segment. Under fluoroscopic control the balloon is expanded with 0.5–1.0 cc dilute arteriographic contrast material. The balloon is then emptied and moved the approximate length of the case segment and reexpanded to gradually dilate the entire stenosed segment. (It is important to use dilute angiographic contrast material to inflate the balloon as undiluted material may occlude the lumen of the balloon cannula. At the end of the procedure this portion of the apparatus should be well irrigated.)

2) For short-shelf or weblike obstructions. After the empty balloon and catheter apparatus are placed above the lesion, the balloon is partially inflated and carefully pulled toward the stenosis. Resistance to the inflated balloon usually indicates the site of stenosis.

After the mild resistance of the stenotic segment is noted the balloon is slightly deflated and positioned in the stenotic segment. The balloon is then expanded with 0.5–1.0 cc dilute contrast material.

Dotter also described an alternative method in which the partially expanded balloon is continuously pulled down until a sudden relief in resistance is noted at the fingertips or visualized under fluoroscopy. Repetition of this procedure as the balloon is increasingly expanded will progressively dilate the stenosed area. The balloon should never be expanded so much that free movement is impossible in the lumen of the nonstenotic portion of the artery.

Intermittent control angiograms should be obtained and the amount of dilatation documented by high-quality comparative angiograms.

Because of the slits in the catheter at the site of the balloon, the material in the catheter, and the balloon itself, there is a great tendency toward thrombus formation. Speed is a factor in prevention. Before initiating the procedure the operator should be mentally prepared for thrombus formation and have appropriate apparatus available for treatment. As soon as dilatation is complete the dilated catheter and balloon should be removed and replaced by a conventional catheter via standard guide wire techniques. A second 3000-U dose of heparin sodium should be injected above the dilated segment as a final maneuver prior to removal of the diagnostic catheter.

Dotter also described use of sulfinpyrazone (Anturane) 2 mg four times a day to inhibit platelet aggregation.

Grüntzig Technique

A catheter system for vascular dilatation introduced by Grüntzig is distinctly different from those previously described. A single catheter apparatus is employed using a balloon dilatation technique rather than a coaxial technique. The balloon is specially designed so that substantial intraluminal pressure can be applied without overexpanding the balloon. Specifi-

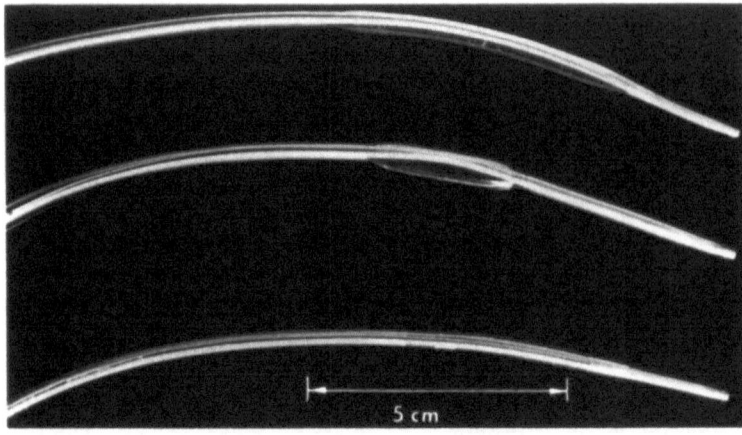

Fig. 106. Catheters for transluminal angioplasty, Grüntzig technique.

cally, internal pressure within the balloon can be maintained at 4–8 atmospheres of pressure without distending the balloon beyond the working outer diameter of 8 mm.

Equipment (Fig. 106)

Two basic catheters 8 F in outer diameter (Schneider Medintag Ag, Bankgesellschaft, Zurich, USCI, USA). The balloon cross-

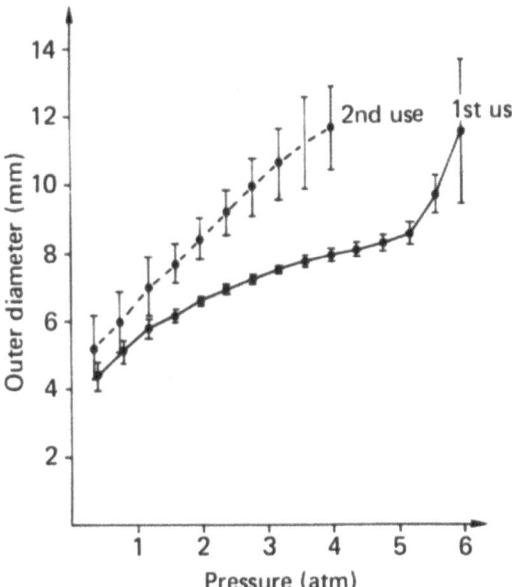

Fig. 107. Grüntzig dilatation catheter. The outer diameter of dilating segments increases with increasing pressure. The temperature is 36.8°C. The iliac artery dilatation catheter has a balloon length of 2 cm and an outer diameter of 8 mm.

sectional diameter of the femoral artery dilatation catheter is 4 mm and the length 4 cm. The balloon cross-sectional diameter of the iliac artery dilatation catheter is 8 mm and the length 2 cm. Similar catheters are manufactured in the U.S. by Cook Incorporated, which provide greater variability in balloon size and length. With continued technological improvement in this field, even better catheters should be available in the future.

Stainless-steel stiffening cannulas 1.2 mm in diameter and 8 cm long

Y adapter

Pressure gauge for balloon

The catheter is constructed so that a thin polyvinyl chloride sleeve fits tightly over its core; it has a single groove to allow passage of air or contrast material. The balloon apparatus is located 4 cm from the tip of the catheter. A unique characteristic of the balloon is that when it is new, inflation up to 6 atm will result in dilatation only to the specified diameter. This characteristic changes, however, with increased use (Fig. 107).

Technique

Superficial Femoral Artery Dilatation. An anterograde puncture is made in the common femoral artery. This can be the most critical part of the procedure from a technical point of view. The puncture must originate quite high on the skin surface to obtain the appropriate level. A 5 F catheter is then introduced into the superficial femoral artery and arteriograms, as well as direct pressure measurements, are obtained.

The 8 F Grüntzig femoral artery dilatation catheter is passed into the superficial femoral artery. In cases of high-grade stenosis, the stenotic area is negotiated by a J wire, if possible, and the catheter passed distal to the area. The balloon is inflated for 15–30 seconds and deflated. Use of a Y adapter attached to the central lumen allows injection of contrast as well, or pressure monitoring while the guide wire remains in place. This device is extremely helpful because, in general, it is not desirable to traverse the diseased area more than once with the guide wire. The dilatation maneuver is repeated, the catheter is withdrawn proximal to the narrowing and the results evaluated by fluoroscopy and arteriography.

When dilatation is successful, no further manipulation is performed, 5000 U heparin is administered intraarterially, and the procedure is terminated. The patient remains in bed until the following morning when ambulation and activity are encouraged.

In patients with superficial femoral artery *occlusions*, the area of abnormality is marked on the field by using fluoroscopy and metallic markers. A .038-inch Teflon straight guide wire is passed through the occlusion. The dilatation catheter is then passed to the most distal part of the occlusion, which is documented by contrast injection through the Y adapter. Segmental inflation of the balloon to 6–8 atm of pressure is monitored under fluoroscopy. Thirty percent or less of dilute contrast is used to distend the balloon. The catheter is withdrawn one balloon length and the process repeated. When adequate dilatation is accomplished, the guide wire may be removed and arteriography performed.

Technique

Iliac Artery Dilatation. A 5 F catheter is introduced into the abdominal aorta from the ipsilateral side of the stenosis and the pressure gradient across the stenosis is documented. If difficulty is encountered in negotiating the narrowing at the time of femoral artery puncture, the 5 F catheter is placed into the external

iliac artery and retrograde arteriography is performed. If preliminary manipulation with the usual J wire and catheterization technique is unsuccessful, a catheter is placed from the contralateral femoral artery to document pressure gradients across the stenosed segment.

The iliac artery dilatation catheter is placed on the side of the stricture (Fig. 108) and a J or straight wire used to traverse the area of stenosis. The balloon is inflated once or twice for 30-second intervals to dilate the stenotic area. The result is evaluated by arteriography via the catheter in the lower abdominal aorta. Pressure gradients are again determined before the examination is completed. Obliteration of pressure gradients rather than morphologic configuration is the end point.

Not uncommonly, large subintimal flaps have remained at least 2–3 years without hemodynamic significance. Angiographically "good-looking" dilatation occurs less frequently in the iliac vessels. These will generally have little significance unless further manipulation is attempted, which could result in immediate occlusion.

Iliac lesions may also be approached from the contralateral femoral artery and with 7 F catheters (Cook Incorporated) from the axillary artery. The approach should be individual-

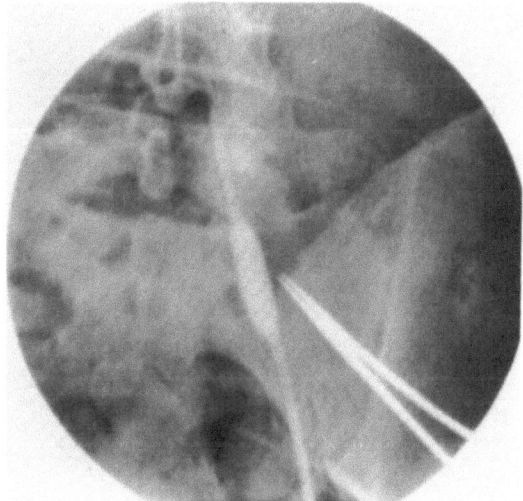

Fig. 108. Grüntzig balloon inflated at the site of left iliac artery stenosis.

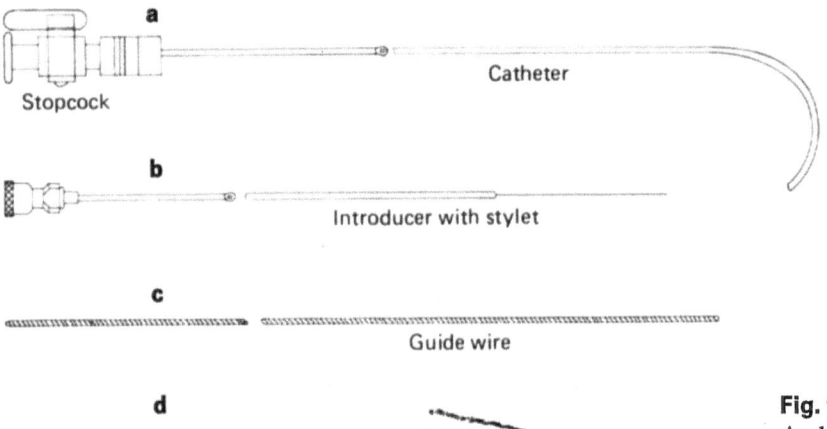

Fig. 109. Gianturco-Wallace-Anderson arterial embolization set.

ized depending upon pathology, age, and anatomic factors.

Heparinization is carried out, and the procedure is terminated. Postangioplasty protocol includes low-dose heparinization for 2–3 days, conversion to salicylate therapy, and follow-up by pulse-volume recording and ankle pressures.

Mechanical Device for Arterial Occlusion

Transcatheter therapeutic embolization, which was described earlier, has had increasing application in the control of hemorrhage from numerous sites and from various causes. For production of complete vascular occlusion or occlusion of a large-caliber vessel, however, embolization with small fragments of clot or Gelfoam is not adequate or desirable. The Gianturco-Wallace-Anderson coil apparatus is effective in permanently occluding medium and large vessels. The apparatus consists of a catheter, introducer with stylet, wire guide, cartridge, and occluding spring embolus [Fig. 109], which can be straightened with the introducer stylet, with attached cotton threads. In an intravascular location the spring regains its shape and the cotton aids in inducing thrombus. The following instructions, developed by Gianturco et al., are taken from the manual provided by Cook Incorporated.

The introducer stylet is inserted into the occluding spring embolus and advanced until the tip of the stylet is flush with the distal tip of the spring embolus [Fig. 110]. Care should be taken to avoid pushing the spring embolus beyond the tip of its cartridge.

To load the occluding spring embolus into the catheter, the distal end of the introducer-cartridge-embolus combination is inserted through the stopcock hub on the catheter [Fig. 111a]. The system should appear as shown in [Fig. 111b].

The introducer is now grasped near the spring embolus [Fig. 111b] and advanced with a slight rotating motion until the spring embolus is pushed from the cartridge into the catheter [Fig. 111c]. Once the spring embolus is outside the cartridge, the latter is withdrawn

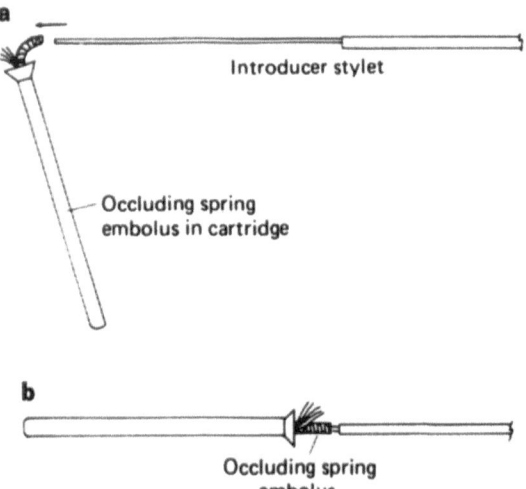

Fig. 110. Insertion of the introducer stylet (**a**) into the occluding spring embolus (**b**).

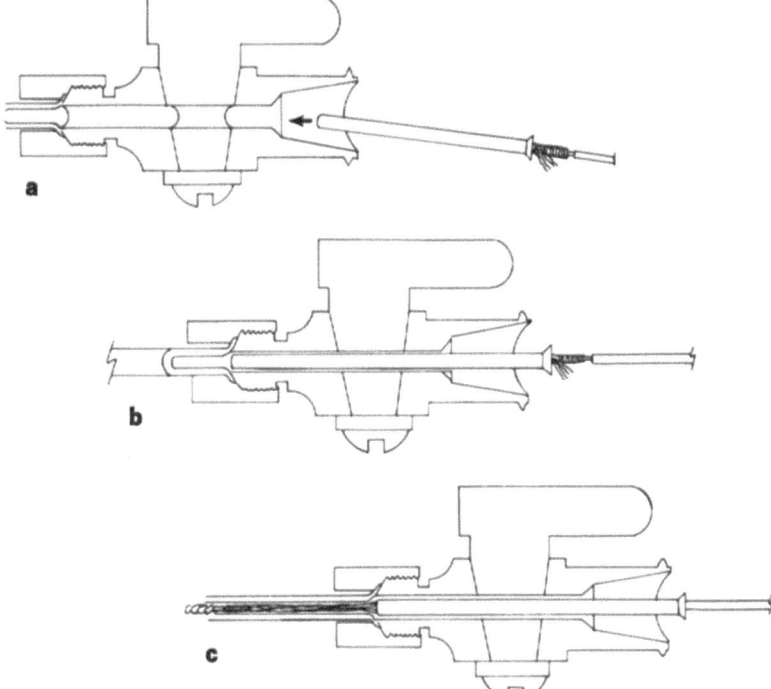

Fig. 111, a–c. Loading the spring embolus into the catheter. **a** The distal end of the introducer-cartridge-embolus apparatus is inserted through the stopcock on the catheter. **b** The introducer is grasped near the spring embolus. **c** It is advanced until the spring embolus is pushed from the cartridge into the catheter.

from the stopcock hub and along the introducer to its hub fitting. The introducer is grasped and used to advance the spring embolus farther into the catheter; they are advanced as far as the length of the introducer will allow. The knob of the introducer stylet is then unlocked from the hub of the outer portion and the stylet is withdrawn until the slight bend in the stylet is visible. The introducer stylet and cartridge are now withdrawn from the catheter, leaving the spring embolus within the catheter.

To eject the embolus from the catheter, the wire guide is inserted into the catheter and advanced until the embolus is pushed free of the distal tip of the catheter where it assumes the configuration shown in [Fig. 112].

If it becomes necessary to replace an occluding spring embolus in its cartridge, the spring is first placed on the introducer stylet, thus straightening the coil. The woolen strands are

straightened and the Teflon cartridge is advanced over the spring embolus until the tip of the spring is near the distal tip of the cartridge [Fig. 113]. To insure that the spring embolus will eject easily from the cartridge, the distal tip of the spring embolus should not be allowed to protrude from the cartridge.

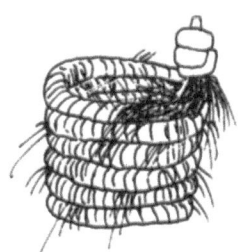

Fig. 112. Spring embolus after ejection from the catheter.

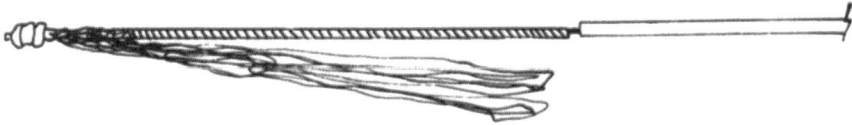

Fig. 113. Replacement of an occluding spring embolus in its cartridge. The cartridge is advanced over the spring embolus until the tip of the spring is near the distal tip of the cartridge.

Interventional Radiographic Procedures in the Urinary Tract

Antegrade Pyelography

Purpose

To provide direct visualization of the upper collecting system and ureters for diagnostic purposes, and in some cases for visualization of the collecting systems for nephrostomy placement

Equipment

22–23-gauge Chiba fine needle
60% contrast
Local anesthesia

Technique

If renal function is adequate, visualization of the upper collecting system may be sufficient to allow performance of antegrade pyelography under flouroscopic control. However, if the kidney is not completely visualized, or if there is a contraindication to the contrast, initial localization of the collecting system may be obtained with ultrasound. This can be done by conventional B-mode scanning with the skin and depth marked prior to moving the patient into the special procedures suite. Recently we have found it extremely convenient to use a real-time ultrasound unit simultaneously with flouroscopy.

Once the upper collecting system is positively identified, a needle pass is planned from the posterolateral approach. Local anesthesia is administered in the usual fashion with a thin 21- or 22-guage spinal needle for adequate deep anesthesia. Antegrade pyelography should be associated with relatively little patient discomfort. The needle is firmly passed toward the collecting system to its final position. After removing the stylet, aspiration using connecting tubing can be performed while the needle is gently withdrawn. Once urine is collected for culture and cytology, if indicated, contrast is injected to the approximate volume of urine

removed. Initial injection of contrast should be gentle, confirming the needle position and anatomic localization. Forceful injection or over-distention should be avoided as intravasation of the infected urine into the vascular system may result in sepsis. When the diagnosis or point of obstruction is uncertain, use of a conventional tilting table may be helpful in placing the distal ureters in a dependent position.

Percutaneous Nephrostomy

Purpose

To provide temporary decompression of an obstructed upper collecting system

Equipment

Multiple side-hole catheters, preferably pigtail in shape, may be used as well as larger caliber nephrostomy sets
22–23 gauge Chiba needle

Technique

Opacification of the upper collecting system is performed by antegrade pyelography. Following visualization of the upper collecting system, an additional puncture may be necessary to obtain a more optimal anatomic access to the upper collecting system. The posterolateral approach is favored in order to provide more renal parenchyma, to give support to the catheter, as well as to avoid the renal hilar structures. Using an 18-gauge polyethylene sheath apparatus (Fig. 114), the kidney and upper collecting systems are punctured from the posterolateral approach. After removal of the trocar, aspiration is continued until the urine is obtained. A .035-inch 3-mm J wire is then passed into the upper collecting system to provide access for catheter exchange. The 18-gauge polyethylene sheath is then advanced into the proximal ureter. Progressive dilatation of the tract, using 6, 7, and 8 French dilators are then performed. Finally, an 8.3

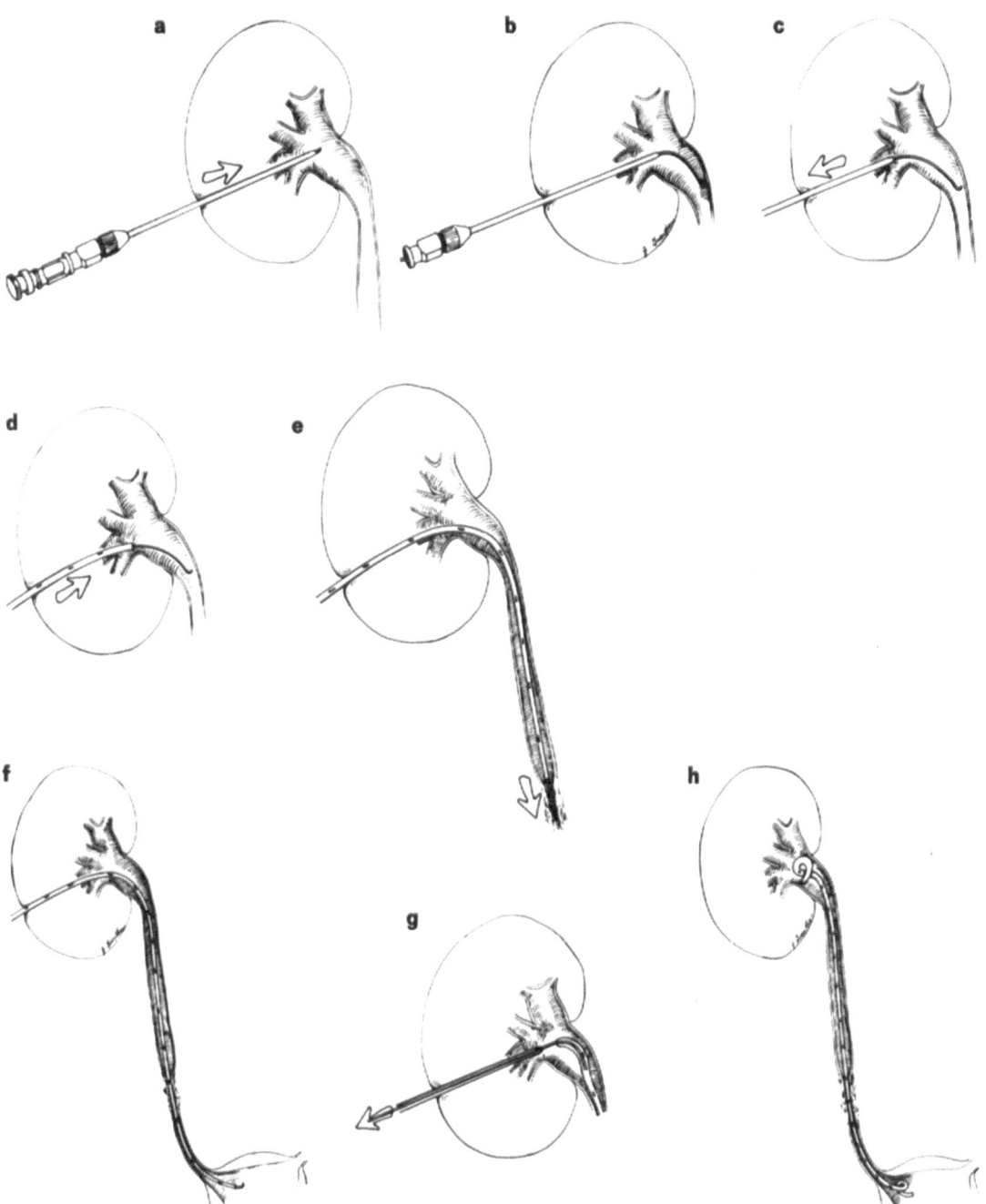

Fig. 114. Percutaneous nephrostomy and stent placement. **a** From a posterolateral approach, the polyethylene sheathed trocar apparatus is advanced into the renal pelvis. **b, c** Following removal of trocar and aspiration of urine, a stainless steel guide wire is passed into the renal pelvis. The catheter may be advanced if it is to be used for drainage, or it may be removed leaving the guide wire in place if a renal stent is to be placed. **d** The stent catheter is passed over the guide wire, and **e** advanced into the ureter towards the point of stenosis. **f** The guide wire is gently advanced through the stenotic area and followed by the catheter. **g** The advancing catheter is removed along with the guide wire once the proximal portion of the stent is confirmed to be within the renal pelvis and the distal portion within the bladder. **h** Following removal of all guide wires and catheters, the stent is in place through the stenosis.

French pigtail angiographic catheter with multiple side holes is exchanged over a guide wire and advanced into the collecting system. The catheter is anchored in place and connected to straight drainage. Additional diagnostic information may be obtained at this time, including urine for cytology.

Complications

Strict attention to anatomic detail will help avoid complications, however, retroperitoneal and renal hemorrhage can still occur and, if significant, may produce alterations in hemoglobin and hematocrit. Brisk, bright red bleeding following initial puncture of the upper collecting system is common and generally self-limited. In patients with long-standing obstruction, appropriate antibiotic coverage may be administered to avoid sepsis. Transient hematuria in association with the nephrostomy placement generally clears within 12 hours. Additional hypothetical complications include perforation of the upper collecting system into the retroperitoneum which, if detected early, may be of little consequence but conceivably may produce urinoma.

Contraindications

Determination of the patient's coagulation state should be made prior to any interventional procedure. Although no absolute contraindications to performance of percutaneous nephrostomy have been identified, severe renal infection, hypertension and bleeding diathesis all add to the possible morbidity of the procedure. These must be weighed against the potential risks in considering the necessity to perform the procedure. A relative contraindication exists in the presence of a bleeding diathesis, and attempts to correct it should be made unless an emergency clinical situation precludes this.

Percutaneous Ureteral Stent Placement

Indications

Percutaneous ureteral stent placement provides long-term internal urinary drainage in the face of ureteral obstruction or stenosis secondary to benign or malignant strictures. Ureteral stents generally have been placed from a retrograde approach via the cystoscope. This is generally done during cystoscopy, when the urologist will also take tissue for histologic study. When placement of a stent is impossible by this method because of obliteration of the ureterovesicle junction, local anatomic deformity or inability to achieve retrograde passage of the stent through the obstruction, the percutaneous method may be helpful.

Equipment

No. 6 or 7 F "double pigtail" silastic ureteral stent (Vance Products)
.035-in. movable J guide wire (3-mm curve).
Diagnostic "cobra" catheter

Technique

Percutaneous stents are generally placed in conjunction with percutaneous nephrostomy (Fig. 114). External drainage allows optimal control of sepsis, infection or other side effects due to the obstruction.

A catheter exchange from the nephrostomy catheter to a cobra-shaped catheter may be performed, using a .035-inch movable core J guidewire. When the wire and catheter are positioned in the renal pelvis, appropriate manipulation of the catheter will enable the operator to enter the ureter. Once the point of obstruction or narrowing is encountered, the core of the guide wire should be advanced, leaving only a minimal curve to the tip of the wire. Since the wire is now rigid, gentle probing with the wire near the obstruction should be employed. Often it may be possible to find the obliterated lumen directly. The wire is negotiated through the obstruction and the catheter is advanced over the wire. The entire assembly is then advanced through the ureteral vesicle junction into the bladder. With the guide wire in the bladder, the catheter is withdrawn and the appropriate stent placed over the wire and advanced as far as possible through the flank. A "pushing" catheter is then placed over the guide wire and used to further advance the stent until the distal pigtail is in the bladder. It is extremely important that the stent lie within the bladder, since future retrieval depends on ready access to the stent via a cystoscope. The pushing catheter is then withdrawn. However, before the guide wire is removed, a new pigtail catheter is placed over the guide wire and advanced to the renal pelvis to provide external drainage for several more days following the stent placement. This allows for other inflammatory debris to drain externally. Before the nephrostomy catheter is removed, a nephrostogram must be performed to insure that there is adequate ureteral drainage and that the stent is working.

Appendix

Treatment of Reactions to Contrast Media

The various procedures described in this text involve administration of contrast material to enhance diagnostic capability. Patients sometimes have adverse reactions to various agents used for contrast. In addition, the invasive nature of the procedures exposes patients to risk. Therefore radiologists involved with these procedures should be able to treat reactions to contrast media and complications related to the invasive procedure itself. They should also have periodic reeducation in cardiovascular support, cardiopulmonary resuscitation, and current drug therapy.

Tables 1 to 7 are reproduced with permission from the manual published in 1977 by the American College of Radiology: *Prevention and Management of Adverse Reactions to Intravascular Contrast Media.* Further reference to this manual is suggested.

As emphasized by the American College of Radiology, radiologists must have knowledge of the classification, manifestations, and severity of possible reactions, a well-formulated plan of action for themselves and their assistants if a reaction occurs, and the necessary medication and equipment readily available for use. Many of these supportive measures may be necessary if complications result from the invasive procedures described in this text.

TABLE 1.   General classification of severe reactions to contrast media, manifestations, and then treatment (American College of Radiology, 1977).

Type	Complication	Treatment

Cardiovascular system	Cardiac arrest:
	  a. Asystole
	  b. Ventricular fibrillation
		a. Sharp blow to precordium
		b. External cardiac massage, etc
		c. External defibrillation, immediately

	Hypotension; syncope	Posture; vasopressors; drugs; etc
	Pulmonary edema	Aminophylline; Demerol; Lasix; phlebotomy; oxygen; morphine
Respiratory system	Respiratory arrest (or obstruction)	Maintain airway (by natural or artificial means) Pulmonary ventilation
Central nervous system	Toxic convulsions	Nembutal or diazepam IV
	Coma	Solu-Cortef IV
"Allergic reaction"	Angioneurotic edema	Adrenaline; Solu-Cortef
	Bronchospasm	Aminophylline; Benadryl

137

TABLE 2. Specific treatment for major reactions to contrast media*
(American College of Radiology, 1977).

Type	Drug	Avg. adult dose	Comments
Cardiac and pulmonary arrest			
Hypotension	Neo-Synephrine IV drip	10 mg in 500 cc IV solution	Oxygen
	Aramine IV drip	5 cc in 500 cc saline (50 mg)	Titrate to Pt's usual BP with IV drip
	Levophed ID	Ampule in 500 cc normal saline or 5% dextrose in water	Trendelenburg position
Hypotension, vasovagal	Atropine IV if indicated	0.5–1 mg IV; repeat if indicated	Often transient and does not require drug; vasopressors not recommended
Bronchospasm	Adrenaline SC	0.1–0.3 cc 1:1000 aqueous	
	Adrenaline IV	0.1–0.3 cc 1:1000 aqueous	Oxygen
	Aminophylline IV	10 cc in 10 min (250 mg)	Give IV slowly
	Solu-Cortef IV	2.0 cc (100 mg)	Give aminophylline slowly
Toxic convulsions	Nembutal IV	0.5 cc q 2 min (25 mg)	Oxygen
	Valium IV	5 mg	May require Solu-Cortef 2.0 cc (200 mg) IV
	Solu-Cortef IV	100 mg	
Pulmonary edema	Oxygen		
	Morphine IV or	10 mg	Elevate upper torso
	Demerol IV	1.0 cc (50 mg)	Venous compression of extremities by rotation tourniquet
	Solu-Cortef IV	2.0 cc (100 mg)	Oxygen
Laryngeal edema	Adrenaline IV	0.3	Endotracheal intubation
		0.1 cc 1:1000 aqueous	May require tracheostomy
	Solu-Cortef IV	2.0 cc (100 mg)	May require additional doses
Hypertensive crisis due to pheochromocytoma	Regitine IV	1.0 cc (5 mg)	

* Modified after Weigen JF, Thomas SF (1958) Reactions to intravenous organic iodide compounds and their immediate treatment. Radiology 71:21.

TABLE 3. What to look for in a serious reaction (American College of Radiology, 1977).

Pallor Diaphoresis Cyanosis Dyspnea Apnea	Signs of hypotension, cardiac arrest, or respiratory arrest
Wheezing Stridor Cyanosis Dyspnea Tachypnea	Signs of bronchospasm, asthmatic attack, or laryngeal edema
Dyspnea Cyanosis Frothy secretions	Signs of pulmonary edema
Cough Headache Dizziness Anxiety Agitation	Usually require no treatment but may be forerunners of more serious reaction

TABLE 4. Minor reactions (American College of Radiology, 1977).

Signs and symptoms	Treatment
Erythema Cough	Observe; no treatment required
Pruritus	Adrenaline 0.1–0.3 cc 1:1000
Urticaria	Benadryl 50–100 mg IV if necessary
Angioneurotic edema Rash	Observe for possible ensuing laryngeal edema
Nausea Vomiting Abdominal cramps	Supportive Ensure patient does not aspirate
Dizziness Light-headedness Sweating	Supportive; reassurance
Headache	Supportive; mild analgesic if necessary
Swelling of salivary glands	Benadryl 50–100 IM; cortisone

TABLE 5. Representative adult drug dosages[a] **(American College of Radiology, 1977).**

Drug	Route	Usual dose	Indication	Comments
Adrenaline 1:1000	SC	0.1–0.3 cc	Allergic reactions, asthma, etc	Acts rapidly; give stat
Adrenaline 1:1000	IV IC	0.2–0.5 cc q.s. 10 cc physiol saline	Asystole in cardiac arrest	Improves cardiac tone; may induce vent fib or change "fine" fib to "coarse" fib
Aminophylline 3¾ grains	IV	250 mg in 10 cc	Bronchospasm, cardiac asthma, pul edema	Inject 10 cc in 10 min slowly! Vasodilation; may cause hypotension
Aramine 1%	IM IV	0.2–1.0 cc 0.1–0.5 cc	Hypotension Profound collapse	Rapid but brief action; titrate to Pt's usual BP
Atropine SO$_4$ 0.6 mg/cc	IV	1.0 cc	Bradycardia, hypotension	Decreases vagal inhibition
Benadryl 1% (10 mg/cc)	IV	3.0–5.0 cc	Allergic reactions	IV antihistamines might cause drowsiness
Calcium chloride 10%	IC	5.0 cc	Asystole in cardiac arrest	Cardiotonic action similar to adrenaline
Demerol 5% (50 mg/cc)	IV	2.0 cc	Pulmonary edema, cardiac asthma	Good analgesic and sedative
Lasix	IV IM	20 mg in 2.0 cc	Pulmonary edema Cerebral edema	Slow injection; separate syringe; rapid diuresis
Nembutal 5% (50 mg/cc)	IV	2.0 cc	Toxic convulsions	Inject slowly; may cause respiratory depression
Regitine	IV	5.0 mg	Hypertensive crisis due to pheochromocytoma	Control by BP
Sodium bicarbonate 3.75 gm/50 cc	IV	50–150 cc	Acidosis in cardiac arrest	Give by slow injection as early as possible; use freely
Solu-Cortef	IV	100–200 mg	Allergic reactions, status asthmaticus, profound collapse	Dose can be repeated
Papaverine	IA	40 mg in 1.0 cc	Arterial spasm	Dilute to 20 cc with physiol saline
Xylocaine 1% (10 mg/cc)	IV	5.0–10 cc	Most cardiac arrhythmias, vent fib	Makes heart more responsive to defibrillation

[a] 1% solution = 10 mg/cc; 2% = 20 mg cc, etc.

IA = intra-arterial   IV = intravenous
IC = intra-cardiac   SC = subcutaneous
IM = intramuscular

Warning: Calcium chloride in the soft tissues may cause a slough. An intracardiac injection of sodium bicarbonate is never given since it will cause endocardial necrosis. Sodium bicarbonate should be used with extreme caution in any patient being digitalized.

TABLE 6.   Doses for urographic and CT studies (American College of Radiology, 1977).

Drug	mg I/ml	Container size (ml)	Total g iodine/ container	Anion	Na:NMG ratio
Small dose (up to 10 g iodine/70 kg adult)—Urographic studies					
Angio-Conray	480	20	9.6	Iothalamate	all Na
Conray-60	282	20	5.6	Iothalamate	all NMG
		30	8.5	Iothalamate	all NMG
Conray-400	400	25	10.0	Iothalamate	all Na
Hypaque 50%	300	20	6	Diatrizoate	all Na
Hypaque 60%	282	20	5.6	Diatrizoate	all NMG
		30	8.5	Diatrizoate	all NMG
Hypaque-M 75%	385	20	7.7	Diatrizoate	1:2
Hypaque-M 90%	462	20	9.2	Diatrizoate	1:2
Isopaque 280	280	20	5.6	Metrizoate	all NMG (with Ca 1.3:59.1)
		30	8.4	Metrizoate	all NMG (with Ca 1.3:59.1)
Renografin-60	288	30	8.6	Diatrizoate	1:6.6
Renografin-76	370	20	7.4	Diatrizoate	1:6.6
Reno-M-60	282	30	8.5	Diatrizoate	all NMG
Reno-M-76	358	20	7.2	Diatrizoate	all NMG
Renovist	372	50	18.6	Diatrizoate	1:1
Vascoray	400	25	10.0	Iothalamate	1:2
Medium dose (10–25 g iodine/70 kg adult)—Urographic studies and CT studies					
Angio-Conray	480	50	24	Iothalamate	all Na
Cardiografin	400	50	20	Diatrizoate	all NMG
Conray-400	400	50	20	Iothalamate	all Na
Conray-60	282	50	14.1	Iothalamate	all NMG
Hypaque 50%	300	50	15	Diatrizoate	all Na
Hypaque 60%	282	50	14.1	Diatrizoate	all NMG
Hypaque-M 75%	385	50	19.3	Diatrizoate	1:2
Hypaque-M 90%	462	50	23.1	Diatrizoate	1:2
Isopaque 440	440	50	22	Metrizoate	47:32 (plus 2.5 Ca and 0.8 Mg)
Renografin-60	288	50	14.4	Diatrizoate	1:6.6
Renografin-76	370	50	18.5	Diatrizoate	1:6.6
Reno-M-60	282	50	14.1	Diatrizoate	all NMG
Reno-M-76	358	50	17.9	Diatrizoate	all NMG
Renovist	372	50	18.6	Diatrizoate	1:1
Renovist II	310	60	18.6	Diatrizoate	1:1
Vascoray	400	50	20	Iothalamate	1:2
Large dose (greater than 25 g iodine/70 kg adult)—Urographic studies and CT studies					
Hypaque 25%	150	300	45.0	Diatrizoate	all Na
Reno-M-DIP	141	300	42.3	Diatrizoate	all NMG
Hypaque-DIU	141	300	42.3	Diatrizoate	all NMG
Conray-30	141	300	42.3	Iothalamate	all NMG

TABLE 7.   Doses for vascular studies (American College of Radiology, 1977).

		Single dose			Total dose			Contrast medium used most frequently
		Small	*Medium*	*Large*	*Small*	*Medium*	*Large*	
Kidney	ml	8	12	15	20	30	45	
	mg I	2.960	4.440	5.550	7.400	11.100	16.650	
Liver	ml	20	35	50	70	120	225	
	mg I	7.400	12.950	18.500	25.900	44.400	83.250	
Spleen	ml	20	40	70	70	120	225	Hypaque 60%
	mg I	7.400	14.800	25.900	25.900	44.400	83.250	Hypaque 75%
Celiac artery	ml	30	45	60	80	120	225	Isopaque 440
	mg I	11.100	16.650	22.200	29.600	44.400	83.250	Renografin-60
Abdominal aorta, venocavography, visceral	ml	30	45	60	80	150	225	Renografin-76 Reno-M-60 Reno-M-76
phlebography	mg I	11.100	16.650	22.200	29.600	55.500	83.250	Renovist I
Pulmonary artery	ml	30	50	60	100	150	200	Renovist II
	mg I	11.100	18.500	22.200	37.000	55.500	74.000	Vascoray
Angiocardiography right heart	ml	35	45	60	90	120	225	
	mg I	12.950	16.650	22.200	33.300	44.400	74.000	
Peripheral arteriography	ml	20	50	80	120	180	240	
	mg I	5.640	14.100	22.560	33.840	50.760	67.680	
Angiocardiography:								
Left heart	ml	30	40	60	70	110	225	
	mg I	11.100	14.800	22.200	25.900	40.700	83.250	Hypaque 75%
Thoracic aorta	ml	40	50	60	90	150	225	Isopaque 440
	mg I	14.800	18.500	22.200	33.300	55.500	83.250	Renografin-76
4 Vessel arch	ml	40	60	80	100	150	225	Vascoray
	mg I	11.280	16.920	22.560	28.200	42.300	83.250	

Note: These doses may be exceeded in special situations.

Table 7 (continued).   Doses for vascular studies (American College of Radiology, 1977).

		Single dose			Total dose			Contrast medium used most frequently
		Small	*Medium*	*Large*	*Small*	*Medium*	*Large*	
Coronary	ml	5	8	10	40 ·	60	225	Renografin-76
arteriography	mg I	1.850	2.960	3.700	14.800	22.200	83.250	
Cerebral angiography:								
Common carotid	ml	8	10	12	16	30	60	
	mg I	2.256	2.820	3.384	4.512	10.152	16.920	
Internal carotid	ml	5	7	9	15	28	45	
	mg I	1.410	1.974	2.538	4.230	7.896	12.690	
External carotid	ml	4	6	8	12	24	40	Conray-60
	mg I	1.128	1.692	2.256	3.384	6.768	11.280	Hypaque 60%
Vertebral	ml	6	8	10	12	24	30	Reno-M-60
	mg I	1.692	2.256	2.820	3.384	6.768	8.460	
Selective spinal,	ml	3	5	12	50	100	225	
bronchial	mg I	0.846	1.410	3.384	14.100	28.200	63.450	
Peripheral	ml	30	60	125		May be repeated		Renografin-60[a]
phlebography	mg I	6.930	13.860	28.880				Renografin-76[a]
								Hypaque 60%[a]
								Hypaque-M 75%[a]
								Hypaque-M 90%[a]
								Conray-60[a]
								Reno-M-60[a]
								Vascoray[a]

[a] Dilute to a 45% solution.
Note: These doses may be exceeded in special situations.

Bibliography

Anticoagulation

Anderson JH, Gianturco C, Wallace S, Dodd G, DeJongh D (1974) Anticoagulation techniques for angiography. Radiology 111:573–576

Hawkins IF, Herbert (1974) Contrast material used as a catheter flushing agent: A method to reduce clot formation during angiography. Radiology 110:351–352

Rizk G, Goodale R, Amplatz K (1973) Vascular endoscopy. Radiology 106: 33–35

Wallace S, Medellin H, deJongh D, Gianturco C (1972) Systemic heparinization for angiography. Am J Roentgenol 116:204–209

Outpatient Arteriography

Giustra PE, Killoran PJ (1975) Outpatient arteriography at a small community hospital. Radiology 116:581–583

The Arterial Puncture

Amplatz K (1962) Percutaneous arterial catheterization and its application. Am J Roentgenol 87:265-274

Desilets DT, Hoffman R (1965) A new method of percutaneous catheterization. Radiology 85: 145–148

Desilets DT, Hoffman RB, Ruttenberg HD (1966) A new method of percutaneous catheterization. Am J Roentgenol 97:519–522

Giustra PE, Killoran PJ (1975) Outpatient arteriography at a small community hospital. Radiology 116:581–583

Judkins MP, Kidd HJ, Frische LH, Dotter CT (1967) Lumen following safety-J-guide for catheterization of tortuous vessels. Radiology 88:1127–1130

Nebesar RA, Pollard JJ (1966) A curved tip guide wire for thoracic and abdominal angiography. Am J Roentgenol 97:508–510

Vitek JJ (1973) Femoro-cerebral angiography: Analysis of 2,000 consecutive examinations with special emphasis on carotid artery catheterization in older patients. Am J Roentgenol 118: 633–647

Percutaneous Axillary Arteriography

Antoine JE, Middleton PJ, Carmody PW (1974) Double catheter technique in aortography. Am J Roentgenol 121:623–635

Beachley MC, Ranninger K (1973) Abdominal aortography from the axillary approach. Am J Roentgenol 119:508–511

Bron KM (1966) Selective visceral and total abdominal arteriography via the left axillary artery in the older age group. Am J Roentgenol 97: 432–436

Glenn JH (1975) Abdominal aorta catheterization via the left axillary. Radiology 115:227–228

Hawkins IF (1972) A deflector catheter approach to the abdominal aorta. Am J Roentgenol 116: 196–198

Kerber C, Mani RL, Bank WO, Cromwell LD (1975) Selective cerebral angiography through the axillary artery. Neuroradiology 10:131–135

Meaney F, Lalli AF, Alfidi RJ (1973) Complications and legal implications of radiologic special procedures. Mosby, St Louis, pp 36–43

Translumbar Aortography

dosSantos JC (1947) Sur la desobstruction des thromboses arterielles anciennes. Acad Chir Bull Mem 73:409

dosSantos R, Lamas A, Periera-Caldos J (1929) Arteriografia de aorta e dos vasor abdominais. Med Contemp 47:93

dosSantos R, Lamas A, Periera-Caldos J (1929) L'arteriographie des membres de l'aorte et de ses branches abdominales. Soc Natl Chir Bull Mem 55:587

Rogoff SM, Lipchik EO. In: Abrams HL (ed) (1971) Angiography, 2nd edn. Vol II. Little, Brown, Boston

Triple-Contrast Bladder Examination

Bartley O, Eckerbom H (1960) Perivesical insufflation of gas for determination of bladder wall thickness or tumors of the bladder. Acta Radiol 54: 241–250

Lang EK, Wishard WN Jr, Nourse MH, Mertz JH (1963) Retrograde arteriography in the diagnosis of bladder tumors. J Urol 89:422–426

Soifer E, Margulies M (1963) Visualization of infiltrating tumors by perivesical gas insufflation. J Urol 89:759–762

Taylor DA, Macker KL, Veenema RJ (1965) A preliminary report of a new method for the staging of bladder sarcoma using a triple contrast technique. Br J Radiol 38:664–672

Intraarterial Use of Lidocaine in Peripheral Angiography

Eisenberg RL, Mani, RL, Hedgcock MW (1978) Pain associated with peripheral angiography: Is lidocaine effective? Radiology 127:109–111

Gordon IJ, Westcott JL (1977) Intra-arterial lidocaine: An effective analgesic for peripheral angiography. Radiology 124:43–45

Wildrich WC, Singer RJ, Robbins AH (1977) The use of intra-arterial lidocaine to control pain due to aortofemoral arteriography. Radiology 124:34–41

The Loop Technique in Visceral Angiography

Mikaelsson CG (1965) Polythene catheter of new shape for percutaneous selective catheterization. Acta Radiol 3:581–591

Reuter SR, Atkin TW (1972) High-dose left gastric angiography for demonstration of esophageal varices. Radiology 105:573–578

Sundgren R (1970) Selective angiography of the left gastric artery. Acta Radiol, suppl 299, 1

Waltman AC, Courey WR Athanasoulis C, Baum S (1973) Technique for left gastric artery catheterization. Radiology 109:732–734

Superselective Angiography

Ayella RJ (1975) An ideal catheter: The simple curve. Vasc Surg 9:147–150

Cope C (1969) A new one-catheter torque-guide system for percutaneous exploratory abdominal angiography. Am J Roentgenol 92:174–175

Dotter CT, Rosch J, Lakin PC, Lakin RC, Pegg JE (1972) Injectable flow-guided coaxial catheters for selective angiography and controlled vascular occlusion. Radiology 104:421–423

Haverling H (1969) Balloon catheters and their percutaneous insertion into the vascular system. Acta Radiol 10:209–217

Jensen R, Olin T (1972) Balloon catheters in angiography. Acta Radiol 12:721–736

Klatte, EC, Sloan OM, Yune HY (1972) Balloon-tip guide for selective and subselective arteriography. Radiology 103:707–709

Komaki S (1976) Simplified superselective catheterization of arterial bleeders. Radiology 118:727–729

Maruyama Y, Wrede D, Van Arsdale E, Sayeg J, Engels EP (1972) Comments on shielding by the lead shot method. Radiology 102:445

Nebesar RA, Pollard JJ (1966) A curved-tip guide wire for thoradic and abdominal angiography. Am J Roentgenol 97:508–510

Nebesar RA, Pollard JJ, Edmunds LH, McKhann CF (1964) Indications for selective celiac and superior mesenteric angiography: Experience with 128 cases. Am J Roentgenol 92:1100–1108

Rabinov K, Simon M (1969) A new selective catheter with multidirectional controlled tip. Am J Roentgenol 92:172–174

Reuter SR (1969) Superselective pancreatic angiography. Radiology 92:74–85

Reuter S (1970) Modification of pancreatic blood flow with balloon catheters: A new approach to pancreatic angiography. Radiology 95:57–63

Rosch J, Grollman JH (1969) Superselective arteriography in the diagnosis of abdominal pathology: Technical considerations. Radiology 92: 1008–1013

Rossi P, Verder CC (1966) The floppy wire as an aid in the catheterization. Am J Roentgenol 97:511

Sammons BP, Neal MP, Armstrong RH, Hager HG (1967) Ten years experience with celiac and upper abdominal superior mesenteric arteriography. Am J Roentgenol 101:345–360

Silverman JF, Castellino RA (1972) Feasibility of a balloon-occlusion technique for obtaining renal interstitial pressure. Radiology 103: 701–702

Takashima T, Yamamoto I, Mitani I, Shin M (1970) Transfemoral superselective celiac angiography. Am J Roentgenol 110: 813–826

Wholey MH, Jackman V (1966) New instrument: Controllable guide for angiography. Am J Roentgenol 97:500–503

Coronary Arteriography

Amplatz K (1963) Technics of coronary arteriography. Circulation 27:101–106

Baltaxe HA, Amplatz K, Levin DC (1973) Coronary arteriography. Thomas, Springfield, Ill

Gensini G, DiGiorgi S (1964) Myocardial toxicity of contrast agents used in angiography. Radiology 82:24–34

Judkins MP (1967) Selective coronary arteriography. I. A percutaneous transfemoral technic. Radiology 89:815–24

Judkins MP (1968) Percutaneous transfemoral selective coronary arteriography. Radiol Clin North Am 6:3

Paulin S, Adams FD (1971) Increased ventricular fibrillation during coronary arteriography with a new contrast medium preparation. Radiology 101:45–50

Sones FM Jr.: Personal communication

Bronchial Arteriography

Ishihara T, Inoul H, Kobayshi K (1974) Selective bronchial arteriography and hemoptysis in nonmalignant disease. Chest 66:633–638

Newton TH, Preger L (1965) Selective bronchial arteriography. Am J Roentgenol 84:1043–1050

Reuter SR, Olin T, Abrams HL (1965) Selective bronchial arteriography. Am J Roentgenol 84: 87–94

Viamonte M, Parks RE, Smoak WM (1965) Guided catheterization of the bronchial arteries. Radiology 85:205–230

Parathyroid Arteriography

Doppman JL, Hammond WG (1970) The anatomic basis of parathyroid venous sampling. Radiology 95:603–610

Doppman JL, Hammond WG, Melson CL, Evens RC, Ketcham AS (1969) Staining of parathyroid adenomas by selective arteriography. Radiology 92:527–530

Jelenko C, Teeslink CR, Herndon JR, Morgan DG, Parrish RA, Moretz WH (1971) Localization of parathyroid adenomata by selective arteriography. Am Surg 37:25–33

Kuntz CH, Goldsmith RE (1972) Selective arteriography of parathyroid adenomas. Radiology 102:21–28

Newton TH, Eisenberg E (1966) Angiography of parathyroid adenomas. Radiology, 86:843–850

Shimkin PM, Powell D, Doppman JL, Marx SJ, Pearson KD, Wells S, Ketcham AS (1972) Parathyroid venous sampling. Radiology 104: 571–574

Venography of the Lower Extremity

Betteman MA, Paulin S (1977) Leg phlebography: The incidence, nature and modification of undesirable side effects. Radiology 122:101–104

Rabinov K, Paulin S (1972) Roentgen diagnosis of venous thrombosis in the leg. Arch Surg 104:133–144

Rogoff SM, DeWeese JA (1960) Phlebography of the lower extremity. JAMA 1972:1599–1606

Pulmonary Angiography

Stein MA, Winter J, Grollman JH (1975) The value of the pulmonary-artery-seeking catheter in percutaneous selective pulmonary arteriography. Radiology 114:299–304

Miller RE (1972) Internal jugular pulmonary arteriography and removal of catheter emboli. Radiology 102:200–202

Glenn JH, Ranninger K (1975) A variation of the technique of transfemoral pulmonary arteriography. Radiology 117:473

Grollman JH, Gyepes MT, Helmer E (1970) Transfemoral selective bilateral pulmonary arteriography with a pulmonary-artery-seeking catheter. Radiology 96:202–204

Westcott JL, Lynch WA (1972) The percutaneous axillary vein approach to selective pulmonary angiography. Radiology 103:551–554

Azygography

Schobinger R, Ruzicka FF Jr (1964) Vascular roentogenology. Macmillan, New York, pp. 486–511

Schwartz (1959) Azygography. Radiology 72:338
Costal intra-osseous venography. (1956) Cleve Clin Q 23:155

Epidural Venography

Drasin GF, Daffner RH, Sexton RF, Cheatham WC (1976) Epidural venography: Diagnosis of herniated lumbar intervertebral disc and other disease of the epidural space. Am J Roentgenol 126:1010–1016

Gargano FD, Meyer JD, Sheldon JJ (1974) Transfemoral ascending lumbar catheterization of the epidural veins in lumbar disk disease. Radiology 111:329–336

Gershater R, Holgate RC (1976) Lumbar epidural venography in the diagnosis of disc herniations. Am J Roentgenol 126:992–1002

LePage JR (1974) Transfemoral ascending lumbar catheterization of the epidural veins. Radiology 111:337–339

Miller MR, Handel SF, Coan JD (1976) Transfemoral lumbar epidural venography. Am J Roentgenol 126:1003–1009

Myelography

Amundsen P, Skalpe IO (1975) Cervical myelography with a water-soluble contrast medium (metrizamide). Neuroradiology 8:209–212

Brinker RA (1973) Lumbar spinal puncture for neuroradiology procedures. Am J Roentgenol Radium Ther Nucl Med 118:674–676

Brinker RA, Vienne GA (1973) Routine positive contrast myelography on the mimer III. Am J Roentgenol Radium Ther Nucl Med 118:695

Chynn KY (1973) Painless myelography: Introduction of a new aspiration cannula and review of 541 consecutive studies. Radiology 109:361–367

Dullerud R, Morland T (1976) Adhesive arachnoiditis after lumbar radiculography with

dimer-X and depo-medrol. Radiology 119:153–155

Heinz ER, Goldman RL (1972) The role of gas myelography in neuroradiologic diagnosis. Radiology 102:629–634

Irstam L, Sundström R, Sigstedt B (1974) Acta Lumbar myelography and adhesive arachnoiditis. Radiology 15:356–368

Peterson HO (1975) The hazards of myelography. Radiology 115:237–239

Skalpe IO, Amundsen P (1975) Lumbar radiculography with metrizamide. A non-ionic water-soluble contrast medium. Radiology 115:91–95

Splenoportography

Leger L (1955) Splenoportography. Masson & Cie, Paris

Panke, Ruzicka FF Jr, Rossi P (1959) Technique, hazards and usefulness of percutaneous splenic portography. JAMA 169:1032

Ruzicka FF Jr, Gould H, et al (1960) Value of splenic Portography in the diagnosis of intrahepatic and extrahepatic neoplasms. Am J Med 29:434

Schobinger R, Ruzicka FF Jr (1964) Vascular roentogenology. Macmillan, New York, pp. 572–612

Seldinger SI (1957) A simple method of catheterization of the spleen and liver. Acta Radiol 48:93

Sialography

Heun YY, Klatte EC (1972) Current status of Sialography. Am J Roentgenol Radium Ther Nucl Med 115:420

Potter GD Sialography and the salivary glands. Otolaryngol Clin North Am

Selective Bronchography

Amplatz K (1970) Lateral decubitus bronchography with a single bolus. Radiology 95:439

Avery ME (1970) Bronchography: Outmoded procedure. Pediatrics 46:333

Fennessey JJ (1966) A technique for the selective catheterization of segmental bronchi using arterial catheters. Am J Roentgenol 96:939

Rossi P, Ruzicka FF Jr (1965) Transtracheal "selective bronchography." Radiology

Sargent EN, Turner F (1968) Percutaneous transcricothyroid membrane. Selective bronchography. Am J Roentgenol Radium Ther Nucl Med

Nelson W, Christoforisis AJ (1973) Bronchography in disease of the adult chest. Radiol Clin North Am

Trapnell DH (1971) Some principles of interpretation of bronchograms, Br J Radiol 42:125

Contrast Laryngography

Fabrikant J, et al (1962) Contrast laryngography in evaluation of laryngeal neoplasms. Am J Roentgenol Radium Ther Nucl Med 87:822–835

Powers WE, et al (1957) Contrast examination of larynx and pharynx Radiology 68:169–177

Jing BS (1970) Roentgen examination of the larynx and hypopharynx. Radiol Clin North Am 8:361–386

Johnson TH Jr (1971) Laryngography: The procedure of choice for benign laryngeal lesions. Am J Roentgenol Radium Ther Nucl Med 3:109–114

Hysterosalpingography

Cameron DD, Stervig MJ, Henry S (1979) Hysterosalpingography using a Foley catheter. Radiology 131:542

Foda MS, et al (1962) Hysterography in diagnosis of abnormalities of the uterus (congenital abnormalities). Radiology 35:115

Fullenlove TM (1969) Experience with over 2000 uterosalpingographies. Am J Roentgenol Radium Ther Nucl Med 106:463–471

Henry GW, Hunter RG (1960) Hysterosalpingography with water soluble medium (salpix). Am J Roentgenol Radium Ther Nucl Med 84:924

Rozin S (1965) Uterosalpingography in gynecology. Thomas, Springfield, Ill

Siegler AM (1967) Hysterosalpingography. Harper & Row, New York

Spruer DB, Wilson RF, Arronet GH (1979) Foley catheter hysterosalpingography—A simplified technique for investigating infertility. Radiology 131:543

Yoder IC, Plister RC (1979) Balloon catheter hysterosalpingography. Am J Radiol 133:335

Gynecography (Pelvic Pneumography)

Abrams BS (1955) Pneumography as an aid in the diagnosis of gynecologic disorders. Am J Obstet Gynecol 70:115

Buice JW (1957) Abdominal and pelvic pneumography. Radiology 69:704

Daves ML, Diner WC, Brenner GH (1964) Pelvic pneumography. Am J Roentgenol 92:390–399

Gershon-Cohen J (1952) Pelvic pneumoperitoneum. X-ray appearance of normal female pelvic organs. Am J Obstet Gynecol 64:184

Lunderquist A (1968) Pneumopelvigraphy in the early diagnosis of intersexuality. Am J Roentgenol Radium Ther Nucl Med 103:202–209

Schultz E, Rosen S (1961) Gynecography. Am J Roentgenol Radium Ther Nucl Med 86:866–878

Stevens GM (1969) Pelvic pneumography. Semin Roentgenol 4:252–266

Lymphangiography

Arts V (1967) An injection apparatus for lymphangiography. Am J Roentgenol Radium Ther Nucl Med 100:466–467

Fischer HW, Zimmerman GR (1959) Roentgenographic visualization of lymph nodes and lymphatic channels. Am J Roentgenol Radium Ther Nucl Med 81:517–534

Herman PG, Benninghoff DL, Nelson JH Jr, Mellins HJ (1963) Roentgen anatomy of the ilio-pelvic-aortic lymphatic system. Radiology 80:182–193

Piver MS, Wallace S, Castro JR (1971) The accuracy of lymphangiography in carcinoma of the uterine cervix. Am J Roentgenol Radium Ther Nucl Med 111:278–283

Schaffer B, Koehler PR, Daniel CR, Wohl GT, Rivera E, Meyers WA, Skelley JF (1963) A critical evaluation of lymphangiography. Radiology 80:917–930

Viamonte M Jr, Parks RE (1964) Progress in angiography. Thomas, Springfield, Ill, pp 521–554

Wallace S, Jackson L, Dodd GD, Greening RR (1965) Lymphangiographic interpretation. Radiol Clin North Am 3:467–485

Wiljasalo M (1965) Lymphographic differential diagnosis of neoplastic diseases. Acta Radiol 247 (suppl): 1–143

Preoperative Localization of Mammographically Demonstrated Nonpalpable Lesions of the Breasts

Berger SM, Curcio BM, Gershon-Cohen J, et al (1966) Mammographic localization of unsuspected breast cancer. Am J Roentgenol Radium Ther Nucl Med 96:1046–1052

Dodd GD (1974) Preoperative localization of nonpalpable lesions. In: Gallagher HS (ed) Conference on detection and treatment of early breast cancer. Wiley, New York, 1974, pp 151–153

Frank A, Hall F, Steer M (1976) Preoperative localization of nonpalpable breast lesions demonstrated by mammography. N Engl J Med 295:259–260

Libshitz H, Feig S, Fetouh S (1975) Needle localization of nonpalpable breast lesions. Presented at the 61st annual meeting of the Radiologic Society of North America, Chicago

Merten C, Wecksell A (1975) Breast biopsy localization by the spot method with water soluble contrast material. Presented at the 61st annual meeting of the Radiologic Society of North America, Chicago

Rosato FE, Thomas J, Rosato EF (1973) Operative management of nonpalpable lesions detected by mammography. Surg Gynecol Obstet 137:491–493

Simon N, Lesnick GJ, Lerer WN, et al (1972) Roentgenographic localization of small lesions of the breast by the spot method. Surg Gynecol Obstet 134:572–574

Stevens GM, Jamplis RW (1971) Mammographically directed biopsy of nonpalpable breast lesions. Arch Surg 102:292–295

Threatt B, Appelman H, Dow R, et al (1974) Percutaneous needle localization of clustered mammary microcalcifications prior to biopsy. Am J Roentgenol Radium Ther Nucl Med 121:839–842

Transhepatic Portal Venography

Gothlin J, Dencker H, Tranberg K (1975) Technique and complications of transumbilical catheterization of the portal vein and its tributaries. Am J Roentgenol Radium Ther Nucl Med 125:431–436

Gothlin J, Lunderquist A, Tylen U (1974) Selective phlebography of the pancreas. Acta Radiolog 15:474–480

Rosch J, Dotter CT (1975) Retrograde pancreatic venography. Radiology 114:275–279

Viamonte M, LePage J, Lunderquist A, et al (1975) Selective catheterization of the portal vein and its tributaries. Radiology 114:457–460

Transjugular Approach to the Liver

Hanafee WN, Rosch J, Weiner M (1970) Transjugular dilatation of biliary duct system. Radiology 94:429–432

Hanafee WN, Weiner M (1967) Transjugular percutaneous cholangiography. Radiology 88:35–39

Rosch J, Antonovic, Dotter CT (1975) Transjugular approach to the liver, biliary system, and portal circulation. Am J Roentgenol Radium Ther Nucl Med 125:602–608

Rosch J, Dotter CT (1975) Retrograde pancreatic venography: Experimental study. Radiology 114:275–279

Rosch J, Hanafee WN, Snow H (1969) Transjugular portal venography and radiologic portacaval shunt: Experimental study. Radiology 92:1112–1114

Rosch J, Hanafee WN, Snow H, Barenfus M, Gray R (1971) Transjugular intrahepatic portacaval shunt: Experimental work. Am J Surg 121:588–592

Rosch J, Lakin PC, Antonovic R, Dotter CT (1973) Transjugular approach to liver biopsy and transhepatic cholangiography. N Engl J Med 289:227–231

Weiner M, Hanafee WN (1970) Review of transjugular cholangiography. Radiol Clin North Am 8:53–68

Screw Needle Apparatus for Obtaining Cytologic Material

Nordenstrom B (1975) New instruments for biopsy. Radiology 117:474–475

Sinner WN (1976) Complications of percutaneous transthoracic aspiration needle biopsy. Acta Radiol (Diagn) 17:813

Nonoperative Extraction of Retained Biliary Calculi

Bean WJ, Smith SL, Mahorner HR (1973) Equipment for non-operative removal of biliary tract stones. Radiology 107:452–453

Burhenne HJ, (1973) Non-operative retained biliary tract stone extraction. Am J Roentgenol Radium Ther Nucl Med 117:388–398

Fennessy JJ, You K-D (1970) A method for the expulsion of stones retained in the common bile duct. Am J Roentgenol Radium Ther Nucl Med 110:256–259

Leary JB, Parshall WA (1972) Percutaneous common-duct stone extraction. Radiology 105: 452–454

Light W (1973) Extraction of residual biliary calculi in x-ray department. J Can Assoc Radiol 24: 209–214

Patterson HC, Grice OD, Bream CA (1973) Overlooked gallstones and their retrieval. Am J Surg 125:257–264

Wendth AJ, Lieberman RC, Alpert M (1972) Non-surgical removal of a retained common bile duct calculus. Radiology 103:207–208

Retrieval of Intravascular Foreign Bodies

Hodel HL (1973) Transfemoral rescue of lost intravascular catheters and guide wires. J Can Assoc Radiol 24:42–46

Juhl B (1973) Percutaneous removal of a catheter-embolism from the right side of the heart. Acta Anaesthesiol Scand 17:37–40

Randall PA (1972) Percutaneous removal of iatrogenic intracardiac foreign body. Radiology 102:591–595

Rossi P (1970) "Hook catheter" technique for transfemoral removal of foreign body from right side of the heart. Am J Roentgenol Radium Ther Nucl Med 109:101–106

Transluminal Angioplasty

Dotter CT (1974) Catheter technics in diagnosing and treating femoral artery atherosclerosis. Geriatrics 29:93–102

Dotter CT, Judkins MP (1964) Description of a new technic and a preliminary report of its application. Circulation 30:654–670

Dotter CT, Judkins MP (1965) Percutaneous transluminal treatment of atherosclerotic obstruction. Radiology 84:631

Dotter CT, Judkins MP, Frische LH, Mueller R (1966) The nonsurgical treatment of ilio-femoral arteriosclerotic obstruction. Radiology 86:871–875

Dotter CT, Rosch J, Anderson JM, Antonovic R, Robinson M (1974) Transluminal iliac artery dilatation—Nonsurgical catheter treatment of atheromatous narrowing. JAMA 230:117–124

Dotter CT, Rosch J, Judkins MP (1968) Transluminal dilatation of atherosclerotic stenosis. Surg Gynecol Obstet 127:794–804

Katzen BT, Chang J (1979) Percutaneous transluminal angioplasty: Technical problems encountered in the first forty patients. Cardiovasc Radiol 2:3–8

Katzen BT, Chang J (1979) Transluminal angioplasty with the Gruntzig balloon catheter. Radiology 130:623–626

Katzen BT, Chang J, Lukowsky G, Abramson EG (1979) A new treatment for renovascular hypertension: Percutaneous transluminal angioplasty. Radiology 131:53–58

Porter JM, Eidemiller LR, Dotter CT, Rosch J, Vetto RM (1973) Combined arterial dilatation and femoro-femoral bypass for limb salvage. Surg Gynecol Obstet 137:409–412

Snyder C, Amplatz K (1973) Nonsurgical treatment of postcatheterization femoral artery occlusion—A new technique. Am J Roentgenol Radium Ther Nucl Med 119:590–596

Zeitler E, Schoop W, Zahnow W (1971) The treatment of occlusive arterial disease by transluminal catheter angioplasty. Radiology 99: 19–26

Mechanical Device for Arterial Occlusion

Gianturco C, Anderson JH, Wallace S (1975) Mechanical devices for arterial occlusion. Am J Roentgenol Radium Ther Nucl Med 124: 428–435

Wallace S, Gianturco C, Anderson JH, Goldstein HM, Davis LJ, Bree RL (1976) Therapeutic vascular occlusion utilizing steel coil technique: Clinical applications. Am J Roentgenol 127: 381–387

Index